# uide

# ...assing OSCEs:

## Candidate Briefings, Patient Briefings and Mark Schemes

### Chief Editor: Zeshan Qureshi

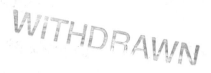

ISBN 9780957149922
Text, design and illustration © Zeshan Qureshi 2013
Chief Editor Zeshan Qureshi
Published by Zeshan Qureshi. First published 2013

Original design (including cover) by Zeshan Qureshi. Page make-up and additonal elements by Natascha Taylor.

A catalogue record for this book is available from the British Library.

Publisher and Chief Editors' Acknowledgements:
I would like to thank all the authors for their hard work, and our distinguished panel of expert reviewers for their specialist input. I am extremely grateful for the support given by medical schools across the UK. I would also like to thank the medical students that have inspired this project, believed in this project, and have helped contribute to, promote, and distribute the book across the UK and the rest of the world.

All images have been taken from 'The Unofficial Guide to Passing OSCEs' 3rd Edition, with the permission of the author. The authors and publishers would like to thank the following for permission to reproduce their images:
Chapter 2, Station 24: David Pottier
Chapter 5, Station 6: Pamela Gulland/Hannah Collinson
Chapter 5, Station 7: Image 1/3: NHS Lothian, Image 2: NHS Fife

A minimum of 50p from each book sale will be reinvested in medical education, or will go to charities, and we are keen to consider charities of YOUR choosing. So far we have raised money for Heart Research UK, Dreamflight, Bluebells Hospice, Madeleine Steel Charitable Trust, Revise4finals, The Shello Orphanage Fund, Alzheimer's Research Trust, The Magic Wand Appeal, Teenage Cancer Trust, and MenCap.

Printed and bound by Cambrian Printers in UK.

# Introduction

## We believe:

**...that fresh graduates have a unique perspective on what works for students.** We have captured the insight of medical students and recent graduates in the language that they used to make complex material more easily digestible *for students*. This textbook has been written by junior doctors and medical students, *but also with the reassurance of review by senior clinicians*

**...that medical texts are in constant need of being updated.** *Every medical student* has the potential to contribute to the education of others by innovative ways of thinking and learning. This book is an open collaboration with you: the readers of the Unofficial Guide to Passing OSCEs have become the writers of this book. You have the power to *contribute* something valuable to medicine. We welcome your suggestions and collaboration on developing this textbook in the future, and our other titles from adding new stations to simply making what we have already *even better*

**...that medical knowledge should be acquired in a fun and memorable way,** *which is why we have made this book practical, so that you can use it in groups to practise with friends when you revise for your OSCEs*

**...that medical knowledge should be spread and shared at a minimal cost to the student.** We will also continue to support medical education projects, through developing the writing skills of our readers.

**...as well, we will continue to support charities of your choosing.** So far money has been donated to Heart Research UK, Dreamflights UK, Alzheimer's UK, Teenage Cancer Trust, Mencap, The Magic Wand Appeal, Bluebells Hospice, Reviseforfinals, and The Shello Orphanage Fund.

*We appreciate that OSCEs are often the most stressful exams you will take at medical school..................*

# The Unofficial Guide to Passing OSCEs:
## Candidate Briefings, Patient Briefings and Mark Schemes

Now in its Third Edition, **The Unofficial Guide to Passing OSCEs** has been received with wide acclaim. **Candidate Briefings, Patient Briefings, and Mark Schemes** is designed to help you practically go through a mock OSCE and structure your OSCE revision. Get into groups, or read through it on your own, and start practising!

**Email:** zeshanqureshi@doctors.org.uk
**Facebook:** http://www.facebook.com/groups/213464185413737/
**Twitter:** @DrZeshanQureshi

*Histories*
**10** Stations

*Examinations*
**25** Stations

*Orthopaedics*
**7** Stations

*Communication Skills*
**10** Stations

*Practical Skills*
**10** Stations

*Radiology*
**3** Stations

*Obstetrics and Gynaecology*
**9** Stations

*Psychiatry*
**8** Stations

*Paediatrics*
**10** Stations

*...This book aims to **empower your examination preparation and help you on your way to excelling in the OSCE.*** We wish you all the best in your upcoming examinations and your future medical career.

*Please get in touch.*

*We look forward to working with you,*

*Zeshan*

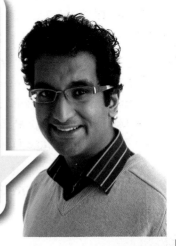

# Authors

**Chief Editor:** Zeshan Qureshi
Paediatric Trainee *(Southampton University)*

**Senior Clinical Editor:** Patrick Byrne
General Medical Physician and GP
*(Belford Hospital Fort William)*

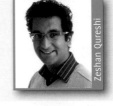 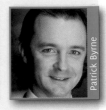

**Obstetrics And Gynaecology:** Matt Wood
Obstetrics And Gynaecology Trainee
*(Southampton University)*

**Radiology:** Mark Rodrigues
Radiology Trainee *(Edinburgh University)*

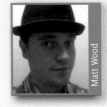 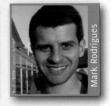

**Histories / Communication Skills:** Matt Harris
Core Medical Trainee *(Southampton University)*

**Psychiatry:** Sabrina Qureshi
Foundation Doctor *(Kings College London)*

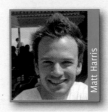 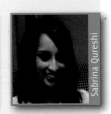

**Examinations:** Lizzie Casselden
Medical Student *(Southampton University)*

**Practical Skills:** Chris Moseley
Foundation Doctor *(Southampton University)*

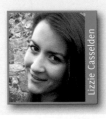 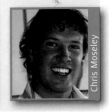

**Orthopaedics:** Chris Gee
Orthopaedic Trainee *(Aberdeen University)*

**Student Reviewer:** Katherine Lattey
Medical Student *(Brighton and Sussex Medical School)*

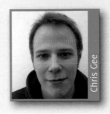 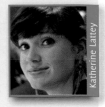

# Table of Contents

## 3. Orthopaedics *(Chris Gee)*

## 4. Communication Skills *(Matt Harris)*

## 5. Practical Skills *(Chris Moseley)*

# 6. Radiology *(Mark Rodrigues)*

# 7. Obstetrics and Gynaecology *(Matt Wood)*

# 8. Psychiatry *(Sabrina Qureshi)*

# 9. Paediatrics *(Zeshan Qureshi)*

# Foreword

*OSCEs are a unique style of examination sat by medical students where structured preparation is the key to success. Nothing can substitute time spent on the wards but an additional revision tool, to help you reach the highest grades, is practising and acting out scenarios (no matter how ridiculous you feel) with another student.*

This book presents a wide range of example scenarios that will ensure that you think in a logical manner and allow you to practise the stations, therefore reducing the anxiety when you perform under assessment. Each station contains instructions for the student, an extensive mark scheme and realistic directions for the patient so that your revision is as similar to the real exam as possible. Using this resource will guide your OSCE revision, enabling you to progress in skill and gain formative feedback. Questions at the end of each station test your knowledge or force you to think logically when giving a sensible suggestion if you're not quite sure!

This book has been written and reviewed by doctors and students who know what medical schools like to examine on, therefore it is a focused, up-to-date and universally applicable resource for the clinical years of training.

*Good luck in your upcoming OSCEs and may you make the very best of your preparation time!*

*Katherine Lattey*
**Medical Student**
**Brighton and Sussex Medical School**

# OSCE Strategy

## Success in exams is due to 5 key things:

1 // Preparation
2 // Practice
3 // Practice
4 // Practice
5 // Practice

*You'll notice that "luck" is not listed. With this in mind,*
*may I recommend some of the following strategy points:*

1 // Know the format of your OSCE: how long do you get per station?
How long do you get to read the brief? *Ask the doctors who sat the*
*exam last year!*

2 // Read the instructions and do exactly what is asked. For example
one year, the cardiac examination candidate briefing stated
'you may assume there is no hepatomegaly'. *Therefore, in*
*this case, don't examine for hepatomegaly!*

3 // The actor is a real patient. Good actors do not act. They inhabit
the role (this is why movies are believable). *Treat them as*
*a real patient.*

4 // Look and act like a doctor. Dress and present yourself
professionally, speak purposefully and confidently, maintain
good posture, and genuinely show interest in the 'patient' and
their problem. *Do a practise run in the clothes you are going to*
*wear!*

5 // Always present your histories and your examinations back to an
examiner – *a colleague or qualified doctor.*

6 // Your technique is more important than "getting" the actual diagnosis. This is because correct technique will lead you to the diagnosis. For example, there is a mark for correct percussion technique. *Most students (and many doctors) fail by not lifting their percussing finger off on their last 'tap'. This error gives a different note and will lead you to misinterpret.*

7 // Do not throw away "easy" marks - things you should be doing automatically. You will see featured on almost every mark-sheet: *introducing yourself, explaining your role, maintaining good eye contact, washing hands.* Do not assume you are doing all of these, or doing them correctly. *Get a colleague to critique you as harshly as possible – much preferable to an examiner doing so.*

8 // Don't get scared or intimidated by the examiner. You get a new one at the end of each station! It is possible to score really high marks overall in your OSCE even if you fail a station: *people that design the OSCEs understand that for a whole host of reasons, one or two stations might not go as well as you deserve them to go.*

9 // Practice 2 minutes of silence after your first question, (or one minute if your OSCE station is short). *Time yourself or be timed and no matter how strong the urge, do not interrupt the patient until 2 minutes are up.* Nothing more than an encouragement to continue (if required). You will get far more information this way and your consultation will actually be quicker as a result.

10 // The marks that seem harder to obtain will come with practice. *When you no longer need to remember which part of the examination comes next, you can focus on the patient, the non-verbal cues such as fear in their voice, or the fact they look exhausted or stressed etc.* This will also mean you can focus on interpreting clinical signs, rather than remembering how to elicit them.

11 // After a little more practise, try and become more and more patient led: *don't have a predefined list of questions to go through in a specific order.* Instead cover topics and patient anxieties in the order they naturally come up in the consultation.

12 // A differential diagnosis is as important as the diagnosis, *if not more so.*

13 // Finally, make sure you always *thank the patient and ensure they are covered up appropriately, maintaining their dignity* before you turn to speak to the examiner.

*Use this book! Go in pairs to examine your patients.* One of you should play the role of examiner using these marksheets: you learn from observing others too. Explain to the patient what you would like to do, and with their permission simulate your exam conditions, especially timing. They may find it entertaining!

*Before you leave, please check that you have not used any terms that the patient doesn't understand, and ask if they have overheard any unfamiliar words that they would like you to explain to them.*

*Patrick Byrne*
GP and Physician in General Medicine
Belford Hospital, Fort William

# How to Use this Book

*This book is designed for convenience to you the student.* Each 'station' is divided into several sections, either for you to study by yourself, or to be divided into three roles: 'the candidate' 'the examiner' and 'the patient'. If there are two people in your group, then dont worry, the patient can 'double up' as the examiner as well.

## Candidate Briefing
These are real life instructions that would be read by the candidate before going into the OSCE Station. You will not be able to ask any questions. Take your time to read it, or have it read to you, and then walk into the 'station' and start performing the task.

## Patient Briefing
These are real life instructions that would be read by the actor playing the patient before going into the OSCE Station. As the patient, pay particular attention to questions and concerns you might have going into the consultation.

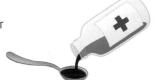

## Examiner Briefing
This is divided into three parts (as follows):

## Mark Scheme
This a check list of things that it is important to cover in the station. This is not based on any specific university mark scheme, but covers the general principles we think are important to cover in the station. The examiner can tick off points as they are covered in the boxes provided, and there is room for the mark scheme to be used five times to gauge progress.

## Questions and Answers for Candidate
These questions can be asked to the candidate. The answers are provided.

## Additional Questions to Consider
These are other questions surrounding the general theme of the station. They are ones to consider and think through as alternatives to those provided.

# Chapter 1

# Histories

# Station 1
# CARDIOVASCULAR HISTORY: CHEST PAIN

*Candidate Briefing: Mrs. Jones is a 60 year-old lady who presented with a two-hour history of central chest pain, shortness of breath and sweating. Please take a history from Mrs. Jones and then present your findings.*

*Patient Briefing: You are 60 years old and your name is Mrs. Jones.*
*You have presented to the emergency department today with a two-hour history of central chest pain. The junior doctor has come to take a history from you.*

The chest pain is central and came on gradually 2 hours ago. The pain is dull in character and radiates to your left arm. The pain came on whilst you were watching television and has not yet gone away. At the moment there is nothing that is making the pain worse although you do not feel like moving. You took some paracetamol earlier but this did not relieve the pain. The pain is eight out of ten in severity.

In addition to the chest pain you are also feeling short of breath and sweaty; both of which have come on over a similar time period to the chest pain. You have no nausea, palpitations, presyncope, syncope, ankle swelling, cough, sputum or haemoptysis.

You are known to have unstable angina and recently you have noticed that your angina pain is coming on with less and less exertion and it has been associated with breathlessness. You did not seek any help for the chest pain and hoped that it would get better again.

You also have high blood pressure and diabetes. You have never had a heart attack, a mini stroke, stroke or problems with circulation in your legs. You have never been told you have high cholesterol.

You take amlodipine 5mg and aspirin 75mg once a day and your diabetes is diet controlled. You have no drug allergies. Your father died of a heart attack aged 50 and your mother has type 2 diabetes. You currently smoke 20 cigarettes a day and have done for the last 40 years. You drink 2-3 glasses of wine every evening. You eat a lot of takeaways and do not eat much fruit or vegetables. You do not do any regular exercise. You are a retired secretary.

*If asked, your main concern is that you are having a heart attack and are worried that you are going to die. You are hoping that the doctor will be able to reassure you.*

# Mark Scheme for Examiner

## Introduction

| Clean hands, introduce self, confirm patient identity and gain consent for history taking | | | | | |
|---|---|---|---|---|---|

## Chest Pain History

| | | | | | |
|---|---|---|---|---|---|
| Site | | | | | |
| Onset | | | | | |
| Character | | | | | |
| Radiation | | | | | |
| Timing and duration | | | | | |
| Exacerbating factors | | | | | |
| Relieving factors | | | | | |
| Severity | | | | | |
| Previous episodes of chest pain | | | | | |

## Associated Symptoms / Systemic Enquiry

| | | | | | |
|---|---|---|---|---|---|
| Shortness of breath | | | | | |
| Autonomic symptoms (nausea, vomiting, sweating) | | | | | |
| Palpitations | | | | | |
| Presyncope and syncope | | | | | |
| Ankle and calf swelling | | | | | |
| Cough and sputum production | | | | | |
| Haemoptysis | | | | | |

## Past Medical History

| | | | | | |
|---|---|---|---|---|---|
| Previous chest pain. Angina or myocardial infarction | | | | | |
| Previous interventions (angiography/CABG) | | | | | |
| Stroke or peripheral vascular disease | | | | | |
| Diabetes mellitus | | | | | |
| Hypertension | | | | | |
| High cholesterol | | | | | |

## Drug History

| | | | | | |
|---|---|---|---|---|---|
| Drug and allergy history | | | | | |

## Family History

| | | | | | |
|---|---|---|---|---|---|
| Family history of heart disease (including age of any significant events e.g. myocardial infarction) | | | | | |

## Social History

| | | | | | |
|---|---|---|---|---|---|
| Smoking status. Duration and quantity of cigarettes smoked | | | | | |
| Alcohol intake, lifestyle (diet, exercise) and occupation | | | | | |

## Finishing the Consultation

| | | | | | |
|---|---|---|---|---|---|
| Elicit patient concerns | | | | | |
| Summarise history back to patient | | | | | |
| Thank patient and close consultation | | | | | |

Histories

## General Points

| Polite to patient | | | | | |
|---|---|---|---|---|---|
| Maintain good eye contact | | | | | |
| Appropriate use of open and closed questions | | | | | |
| Presentation of case | | | | | |

## Questions And Answers for Candidate

### With a convincing history, what ECG changes would support immediate percutaneous coronary intervention?

- With a convincing history, I would be concerned by ST elevation of 1mm or more in consecutive limb leads (I, II, III, aVF, aVL, aVR); or ST elevation of 2mm or more in consecutive chest leads, or new onset left bundle branch block (though some centres are now using ST elevation of 1mm in the limb leads as the criteria for PCI)

### What artery supplies the sinoatrial tissue of the heart?

- The right coronary artery supplies the sinoatrial nodal artery 60% of the time, the remaining 40% of the time it is supplied by the left circumflex artery

## What areas of the heart are supplied by the left anterior descending artery?

- The left anterior descending artery supplies the anterolateral myocardium, the apex and the interventricular septum. Typically it supplies up to 55% of the left ventricle

**?**

## Additional Questions to Consider

1 // What is the differential diagnosis of chest pain?

2 // How might you differentiate the pain of an MI from pericarditis on history?

3 // What are the immediate and later complications of myocardial infarction?

4 // What is the role of primary angioplasty in acute myocardial infarction?

5 // What advice would you give this patient on discharge?

6 // According to current recommendations, what drugs should be on a patient's discharge letter post acute MI?

7 // What groups of people are at higher risk of a silent myocardial infarction?

# Station 2
# RESPIRATORY HISTORY: PRODUCTIVE COUGH

*Candidate Briefing: Mr. Gordon is a 60-year-old gentleman who presents with a 3-day history of a productive cough and has been finding it increasingly difficult to sleep and get around his house. He is a lifelong cigarette smoker. Please take a history from Mr. Gordon and present your findings.*

*Patient Briefing: You are 60 years old and you are called Mr. Gordon. You have presented to hospital with a three-day history of a productive cough. You have been finding it increasingly difficult to sleep and get around your house because of breathlessness.*

Your cough started three days ago and has been getting gradually worse. You are now having severe coughing bouts eight times a day and producing sputum each time. You estimate that you are producing two cupfuls of sputum a day. Your sputum is yellow / green in colour and is thick in consistency. You have not coughed up any blood.

You have been feeling increasingly short of breath over the last three days which came on relatively quickly. You are now breathless at rest and you also feel "wheezy". You can normally walk about 400 yards on the flat before you become breathless.

You have also been experiencing chest pain for the last two days. The pain is in the right side of your chest and is sharp in character. The pain does not move anywhere else, it is constant but is worse when you take a deep breath. It has been relieved slightly by taking paracetamol. At worst it is a six out of ten in severity. You normally have some mild ankle swelling which has not changed recently. You have lost 3kg of weight in the last two months.

You were diagnosed with COPD five years ago and take inhalers for this. You have never needed hospital admission for your COPD before. You have never had tuberculosis or a DVT. You do not know what a pulmonary embolism is but you have never had a clot on the lungs. Regarding medications you use a tiotropium inhaler once a day and a salbutamol inhaler when you need to. You have no drug allergies. Your father was a lifelong smoker and suffered from chronic bronchitis.

You are also a lifelong cigarette smoker. You have smoked approximately 20 cigarettes a day for the last 50 years. You have not had any recent travel. You no longer work but used to be an IT consultant. You have never been exposed to asbestos. You drink 5 pints of alcohol a week and do not keep any pets.

*Your main concern is that you are becoming increasingly reliant on your wife for help with general day to day activities and feel that you are struggling at home.*

# Mark Scheme for Examiner

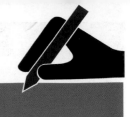

## Introduction

| | | | | | |
|---|---|---|---|---|---|
| Clean hands, introduce self, confirm patient identity and gain consent for history taking | | | | | |

## Cough

| | | | | | |
|---|---|---|---|---|---|
| Duration, character and frequency | | | | | |
| Sputum production and frequency | | | | | |
| Sputum colour, volume and consistency | | | | | |
| Haemoptysis (volume and frequency) | | | | | |

## Shortness of Breath

| | | | | | |
|---|---|---|---|---|---|
| Duration | | | | | |
| Speed of onset | | | | | |
| Exacerbating/relieving factors | | | | | |
| Usual exercise tolerance (how far can they walk on the flat?) and current exercise tolerance | | | | | |
| Orthopnea | | | | | |
| Paroxysmal nocturnal dyspnea | | | | | |

## Associated symptoms/Systemic Enquiry

| | | | | | |
|---|---|---|---|---|---|
| Chest pain (SOCRATES assessment) | | | | | |
| Wheeze | | | | | |
| Ankle swelling | | | | | |
| Weight loss | | | | | |
| Stridor | | | | | |
| Temperature / rigors / night sweats | | | | | |

The Unofficial Guide to Passing OSCEs: *Candidate Briefings, Patient Briefings and Mark Schemes*

## Past Medical History

| | | | | | |
|---|---|---|---|---|---|
| Previous breathlessness and investigations | | | | | |
| Asthma/COPD (including disease control, previous admissions to hospital and ITU) | | | | | |
| Tuberculosis | | | | | |
| DVT/PE | | | | | |
| Chest trauma/Operations | | | | | |
| Malignancy | | | | | |

## Drug History

| | | | | | |
|---|---|---|---|---|---|
| Drug history (including inhalers, courses of steroids and antibiotics) and allergies | | | | | |

## Family History

| | | | | | |
|---|---|---|---|---|---|
| Family history of respiratory disease and atopic illness | | | | | |

## Smoking History

| | | | | | |
|---|---|---|---|---|---|
| Smoking status (including duration and quantity of cigarettes in the past) | | | | | |

## Social History

| | | | | | |
|---|---|---|---|---|---|
| Recent travel | | | | | |
| Occupation and any exposure to asbestos in lifetime | | | | | |
| Pets | | | | | |
| Alcohol intake | | | | | |

Histories

## Finishing the Consultation

| | | | | | |
|---|---|---|---|---|---|
| Elicit patient concerns | | | | | |
| Summarise history back to patient | | | | | |
| Thank patient and close consultation | | | | | |

## General Points

| | | | | | |
|---|---|---|---|---|---|
| Polite to patient | | | | | |
| Maintain good eye contact | | | | | |
| Appropriate use of open and closed questions | | | | | |
| Presentation of case | | | | | |

## Questions And Answers for Candidate

**Classify the causes of pleural effusion and list two causes in each category.**

- Transudative and exudative pleural effusions
- Transudative – cardiac failure, renal failure, hepatic failure, hypothyroid, Meigs' syndrome
- Exudative – pneumonia, pancreatitis, malignancy (primary or secondary) TB, trauma, abscess, connective tissue diseases e.g. rheumatoid arthritis, SLE

## List 3 common bacteria associated with community acquired pneumonia?

- Strep pneumoniae
- Mycoplasma pneumoniae
- Staph aureus
- Haemophilus influenzae

## Which cancer is most associated with asbestos exposure?

- Malignant mesothelioma

## Additional Questions to Consider

1 // Can you list some of the red flag symptoms that would raise your suspicion of possible lung cancer?

2 // Which type of asbestos fibre is considered the most carcinogenic?

3 // List 5 possible causes of haemoptysis

4 // List 2 occupational lung diseases

5 // List 2 lung diseases caused by exposure to animals

6 // List 5 causes of lung fibrosis. (Supplemental question: can you classify this further into causes of upper zone fibrosis and lower zone fibrosis?)

# Station 3
# GI HISTORY: ABDOMINAL PAIN

*Candidate Briefing: Mrs. Smith is a 25-year-old patient complaining of abdominal pain and vomiting. Please take a history from Mrs. Smith and present your findings.*

*Patient Briefing: You are 25 years old and your name is Mrs. Smith. You have presented to hospital with abdominal pain and vomiting.*

You were completely well until two days ago when you started to develop abdominal pain. The pain is on the right side in your lower abdomen. The pain came on suddenly and is sharp in nature; however it doesn't move around your abdomen. The pain is constant and has been getting gradually worse. The pain is made worse if you move around and is better if you stay still. At worst the pain is 8/10 in severity. You have never had this type of pain.

You currently do not feel like eating but your weight has been stable recently. You are feeling sick and have been vomiting for the last 12 hours. You have vomited 4 times but there has not been any blood. You have not had any problems with swallowing. Your bowels have been normal and you last opened them yesterday. You do not know what the word jaundice means but your skin has not turned yellow. You have not experienced any urinary frequency, dysuria or haematuria. You have had no vaginal discharge, bleeding or pain on intercourse (not that you've been trying and with the pain at present you are not remotely interested in finding out). Your last menstrual period was 7 weeks ago.

You have no significant medical or surgical history, except recurrent episodes of chlamydia infection which have required multiple courses of antibiotics. You are not taking any regular medications and do not have any allergies. There is no significant family history. You have never smoked and drink 1-2 glasses of wine a night. You have not had any recent travel and do not know anybody else who has had similar symptoms.

*Your main concern is that you think you might have appendicitis and are worried you might need an operation. You hope the doctor will be able to tell you what he thinks is wrong with you.*

The Unofficial Guide to Passing OSCEs: *Candidate Briefings, Patient Briefings and Mark Schemes*

Histories

# Mark Scheme for Examiner

## Introduction

| | | | | | |
|---|---|---|---|---|---|
| Clean hands, introduce self, confirm patient identity and gain consent for history taking | | | | | |

## Abdominal Pain History

| | | | | | |
|---|---|---|---|---|---|
| Site | | | | | |
| Onset | | | | | |
| Character | | | | | |
| Radiation | | | | | |
| Timing, frequency of pain and duration | | | | | |
| Exacerbating factors | | | | | |
| Relieving factors | | | | | |
| Severity | | | | | |

## Associated Symptoms

| | | | | | |
|---|---|---|---|---|---|
| Anorexia and weight loss | | | | | |
| Nausea, vomiting (including haematemesis and bilious vomiting), abdominal distension | | | | | |
| Dysphagia | | | | | |
| Dyspepsia | | | | | |
| Change in bowel habit (frequency and consistency of bowel motions) | | | | | |
| Blood or mucus per rectum | | | | | |
| Jaundice | | | | | |
| Urological symptoms (frequency, dysuria, haematuria) | | | | | |

| Gynaecological symptoms (vaginal discharge, bleeding, dyspareunia) | | | | | |
| --- | --- | --- | --- | --- | --- |
| Last menstrual period | | | | | |

## Past History

| Past medical history (including previous abdominal pain and investigations) | | | | | |
| --- | --- | --- | --- | --- | --- |
| Past surgical history | | | | | |

## Drug History

| Drug history | | | | | |
| --- | --- | --- | --- | --- | --- |
| Allergy history | | | | | |

## Family History

| Family history (e.g. inflammatory bowel disease, coeliac disease) | | | | | |
| --- | --- | --- | --- | --- | --- |

## Social History

| Smoking history | | | | | |
| --- | --- | --- | --- | --- | --- |
| Alcohol history | | | | | |
| Recent travel | | | | | |
| Contact with infectious sources (e.g. family, friends) | | | | | |

## Finishing the Consultation

| Elicit patient concerns | | | | | |
| --- | --- | --- | --- | --- | --- |
| Summarise history back to patient | | | | | |
| Thank patient and close consultation | | | | | |

Histories

## General Points

| | | | | |
|---|---|---|---|---|
| Polite to patient | | | | |
| Maintain good eye contact | | | | |
| Appropriate use of open and closed questions | | | | |
| Presentation of case | | | | |

## Questions And Answers for Candidate

### If this patient's LMP was 7-weeks late, what tests would you perform?

• Pregnancy test or urinary beta-hCG

### What are the common causes of acute pancreatitis in the UK?

• The commonest causes of acute pancreatitis in the UK are gallstones, ethanol and trauma (be it iatrogenic – ERCP, or blunt trauma e.g. handlebar injuries)

> ## Can you list the structures found in the transpyloric plane (L1)?
>
> - Lumbar vertebra L1, spinal cord (and upper part of the conus medullaris)
> - Origin of superior mesenteric artery from the aorta, termination of superior mesenteric vein
> - Pylorus of the stomach, 1st part of duodenum & duodenojejunal flexure
> - Fundus of the gallbladder, neck and body of the pancreas
> - Spleen
> - Upper pole of the right kidney and hilum of the left kidney
> - Left and right colic flexures

## Additional Questions to Consider

1 // Give five differential diagnoses you would include as causes of an acute abdomen.

2 // List three causes of haematemesis.

3 // Relating to hernias, what is the difference between incarceration and strangulation?

4 // Please tell me some of the radiological findings in small bowel obstruction.

5 // What are the causes of large bowel obstruction?

6 // What is a volvulus and how is it managed?

7 // Define intussusseption.

8 // What is a Meckel's diverticulum?

9 // What is a Richter's hernia?

# Station 4
# GI HISTORY: DIARRHOEA

*Candidate Briefing: Mrs. Sanderson is a 60-year-old lady who has been experiencing severe abdominal pain and diarrhoea for the last 4 days. She was recently discharged from hospital following an appendicectomy. Please take a history from Mrs. Sanderson and present your findings.*

*Patient Briefing: You are 60 years old and your name is Mrs. Sanderson. You have been experiencing severe abdominal pain and diarrhoea for the last 4 days. You were recently discharged from hospital following an appendicectomy.*

You were initially well but then started to develop diarrhoea and abdominal pain four days ago. You are opening your bowels up to eight times a day including at night. Your motions are liquid, foul-smelling and green in colour. There is no blood or mucus that you have noticed. The diarrhoea doesn't have any exacerbating or relieving factors. Sometimes you feel that you won't make the toilet in time to open your bowels. You don't feel like you need to open your bowels again just after opening them.

The abdominal pain is central and came on gradually. It is "crampy" in nature and moves around your abdomen. The pain started a few hours before you started having diarrhoea and comes and goes lasting up to an hour at a time. The pain is worse after eating and is relieved by opening your bowels. At worst the pain is 7 out of 10. You have not had this type of pain before, and it is different to the pain experienced leading up to your appendicectomy.

You currently have little appetite however your weight has been stable. You have been feeling nauseous and feverish but have not vomited. You have not had any swallowing difficulties, indigestion or yellow discoloration of the skin. You have not had any problems passing urine. There is no blood in your urine and no vaginal discharge, bleeding or pain on intercourse. You no longer have periods.

Apart from the recent appendicectomy you have been well with no medical problems or previous operations. You do not take any medications and have no allergies; however you were given a week's course of clindamycin whilst you were in hospital for your appendicectomy. There is no significant family history. You have never smoked and do not drink alcohol. You have not had any recent travel or been in contact with anyone else with similar symptoms.

*Your main concern is that there has been a complication from your appendicectomy and that you are going to need a further operation. You hope the doctor will be able to explain what is going on.*

# Mark Scheme for Examiner

## Introduction

| | | | | | |
|---|---|---|---|---|---|
| Clean hands, introduce self, confirm patient identity and gain consent for history taking | | | | | |

## Diarrhoea History

| | | | | | |
|---|---|---|---|---|---|
| Duration | | | | | |
| Frequency (including nocturnal diarrhoea) and timing | | | | | |
| Consistency: difficult to flush? | | | | | |
| Volume | | | | | |
| Colour | | | | | |
| Presence of blood or mucus | | | | | |
| Exacerbating factors | | | | | |
| Relieving factors | | | | | |
| Urgency, tenesmus | | | | | |

## Abdominal Pain History

| | | | | | |
|---|---|---|---|---|---|
| Site | | | | | |
| Onset | | | | | |
| Character | | | | | |
| Radiation | | | | | |
| Timing, frequency of pain and duration | | | | | |
| Exacerbating factors (e.g. movement, food) | | | | | |
| Relieving factors (e.g. position, medication) | | | | | |
| Severity | | | | | |
| Previous episodes of abdominal pain | | | | | |

Histories

The Unofficial Guide to Passing OSCEs: *Candidate Briefings, Patient Briefings and Mark Schemes*

## Associated Symptoms

| | | | | | |
|---|---|---|---|---|---|
| Anorexia and weight loss | | | | | |
| Nausea and vomiting (including haematemesis and bilious vomiting), abdominal distension | | | | | |
| Dysphagia | | | | | |
| Dyspepsia | | | | | |
| Jaundice | | | | | |
| Urological symptoms (frequency, dysuria, haematuria) | | | | | |
| Gynaecological symptoms (PV discharge, bleeding, dyspareunia) | | | | | |
| Last menstrual period | | | | | |

## Past History

| | | | | | |
|---|---|---|---|---|---|
| Past medical history | | | | | |
| Past surgical history | | | | | |

## Drug History

| | | | | | |
|---|---|---|---|---|---|
| Drug history (including recent medication changes, courses of treatment such as antibiotics) and allergies | | | | | |

## Family History

| | | | | | |
|---|---|---|---|---|---|
| Family history | | | | | |

## Social History

| | | | | | |
|---|---|---|---|---|---|
| Smoking and alcohol history | | | | | |
| Recent travel, and contact with infectious sources | | | | | |

## Finishing the Consultation

| | | | | |
|---|---|---|---|---|
| Elicit patient concerns | | | | |
| Summarise history back to patient | | | | |
| Thank patient and close consultation | | | | |

## General Points

| | | | | |
|---|---|---|---|---|
| Polite to patient | | | | |
| Maintain good eye contact | | | | |
| Appropriate use of open and closed questions | | | | |
| Presentation of case | | | | |

## Questions And Answers for Candidate

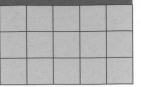

### Can you classify the types of diarrhoea?

- Inflammatory – where there is irritation of the mucosa – e.g. ulcerative colitis
- Secretory e.g. due to infection – there is active secretion of intestinal fluid (e.g. E. coli diarrhoea)
- Osmotic – where the mucosa acts as a semi-permeable membrane – typically with the administration of some types of laxatives
- Increased gut motility – e.g. irritable bowel syndrome

### Where do you biopsy to diagnose coeliac disease?

- 2nd part of the duodenum

## What is a fistula?

- A fistula is an abnormal communication between two eplithelial structures

## Additional Questions to Consider

1 // List 4 causes of altered bowel habit.

2 // List 3 causes of bloody diarrhoea.

3 // Can you list some histological and gross pathological features that distinguish Crohn's disease from ulcerative colitis?

4 // What features of ulcerative colitis lead to an increased risk of cancer developing?

5 // What disease immunosuppressant agents are used in inflammatory bowel disease?

6 // Can you name a monoclonal antibody used in the treatment of inflammatory bowel disease?

7 // What are the histological features commonly seen in biopsy for coeliac disease?

8 // How is coeliac disease best treated?

9 // What are the common sites for colon cancer?

10 // Can you describe a classification system for colon cancer?

# Station 5
# NEUROLOGICAL HISTORY: HEADACHE

*Candidate Briefing: You are the junior doctor on call and have been asked to review Mrs. Heart, a 25-year-old patient who has presented to the emergency department with a new and severe headache. Please take a focused history and present your findings.*

*Patient Briefing: You are 25 years old and your name is Mrs. Heart. You have presented to the emergency department with a headache.*

The headache started six hours ago and is mainly at the back of your head. It came on gradually and is aching in character. The headache does not move anywhere else and has remained constant. The headache does not seem to be made worse by anything although all you want to do is shut your eyes and lie down. The headache is 9/10 severity. You have had no head injury and never had a headache like this before.

You are finding it very difficult to look at bright lights but have not had any changes to your vision or hearing. You report that your neck feels stiff and you are unable to move it. You have also been feeling feverish and generally unwell but have not noticed any rashes. You feel nauseous but have not vomited since the headache began. You have not experienced any light-headedness, dizziness or passed out. You have not noticed any tearing, nasal congestion, altered sensation or weakness. You did not have any symptoms prior to the headache.

You are normally fit and well with no past medical history. You do not take any regular medication and have no allergies. There is no significant family history. You have never smoked but you do drink about a bottle of wine a week. You normally work as a secretary in an office. You have not come into contact with anyone else that is unwell but have heard on the news about an outbreak of meningococcal meningitis in the community.

*Your main concern is that you have meningitis after hearing about the outbreak on the news. You hope that the doctor will be able to do some tests and start you on the right antibiotics.*

## Mark Scheme for Examiner

## Introduction

| | | | | | |
|---|---|---|---|---|---|
| Clean hands, introduce self, confirm patient identity and gain consent for history taking | | | | | |

## Headache History

| | | | | | |
|---|---|---|---|---|---|
| Site | | | | | |
| Onset | | | | | |
| Character | | | | | |
| Radiation | | | | | |
| Timing and duration | | | | | |
| Exacerbating factors | | | | | |
| Relieving factors | | | | | |
| Severity | | | | | |
| History of head injury | | | | | |

## Associated Symptoms

| | | | | | |
|---|---|---|---|---|---|
| Syncope or seizures | | | | | |
| Dizziness | | | | | |
| Loss of consciousness | | | | | |
| Visual or hearing disturbance | | | | | |
| Lacrimation, nasal congestion | | | | | |
| Scalp tenderness | | | | | |
| Altered sensation | | | | | |
| Weakness or change in gait | | | | | |
| Meningism (neck stiffness, photophobia) | | | | | |

| Fever | | | | |
|---|---|---|---|---|
| Rash | | | | |
| Nausea or vomiting | | | | |
| Preceding aura | | | | |

## Past Medical History

| Previous episodes of headache, including investigations | | | | |
|---|---|---|---|---|
| Migraine, TIA, stroke, hypertension, kidney disease, heart problems | | | | |

## Drug History

| Drug and allergy history | | | | |
|---|---|---|---|---|

## Family History

| Family history | | | | |
|---|---|---|---|---|

## Social History

| Smoking and alcohol history | | | | |
|---|---|---|---|---|
| Occupation | | | | |

## Finishing the Consultation

| Elicit patient concerns | | | | |
|---|---|---|---|---|
| Summarise history back to patient | | | | |
| Thank patient and close consultation | | | | |

The Unofficial Guide to Passing OSCEs: *Candidate Briefings, Patient Briefings and Mark Schemes*

## General Points

| | | | | | |
|---|---|---|---|---|---|
| Polite to patient | | | | | |
| Maintain good eye contact | | | | | |
| Appropriate use of open and closed questions | | | | | |
| Presentation of case | | | | | |

## Questions And Answers for Candidate

### What are the common bacterial causes of meningitis in the UK?

- Neisseria meningitidis and strep pneumoniae (80% cases)
- In neonates and premature babies – group B strep and E coli
- In children the 3rd place is haemophilus influenzae B (where vaccination is not offered)
- Listeria monocytogenes is increased in people over 50 but neisseria and strep pneumoniae are still the more common

### What features in the history would raise suspicion of a space occupying lesion?

- Known malignancy or immunosuppression
- Early morning headaches (or a headache that wakes the patient from sleep)
- Early morning vomiting or effortless vomiting
- Headache that is worse lying down and relieved by sitting up

> What would you suspect in a patient presenting with headache, worst early morning or with coughing, sometimes associated with vomiting, and a bitemporal hemianopia?

- Pituitary tumour

## Additional Questions to Consider

**1 //**  What features in the history would suggest migraine as a possible cause?

**2 //**  What types of migraine do you know of?

**3 //**  How might you treat migraine?

**4 //**  What is temporal arteritis (or giant cell arteritis)?

**5 //**  What is idiopathic intracranial hypertension and how does it present?

**6 //**  What is normal pressure hydrocephalus, and what is the triad of presenting symptoms?

**7 //**  What is cryptococcus? What stain is used to find it? What underlying disease is suggested by finding this in the CSF?

# Station 6
# INTERMITTENT CLAUDICATION

*Candidate Briefing: Mr. Brown is a 63-year-old gentleman who presents with worsening leg pain on exertion. He is a long-term cigarette smoker and has type 2 diabetes, with a recent HbA1c of 75mmol/mol. Please take a history from Mr. Brown and present your findings.*

*Patient Briefing: You are 63 years old and your name is Mr. Brown. You have presented to the clinic with worsening left leg pain on exertion. The pain is in the back of your leg and predictably comes on after walking about 30 metres. The pain is a cramping type of pain and does not move anywhere else in the leg. You do not experience this pain at rest or at night. The only thing that seems to bring the pain on is walking and it is only relieved after you rest it for five minutes and take paracetamol. At its worst the pain has been 6/10 in severity. You have been having pain in your left leg for the last 4 months but recently it has been occurring at shorter distances than before.*

You have not had any problems with foot ulcers, changes in sensation or reduced temperature in the legs. Your muscle power feels normal. You have not been experiencing any difficulties with maintaining an erection.

You have tablet controlled type 2 diabetes and a recent HbA1c was elevated at 75mmol/mol. You have not been told that you have high blood pressure or high cholesterol. You have never had an irregular heart beat, any heart disease, strokes or problems with circulation in the legs. You have not had any investigations for this pain and you have not had any operations in the past.

You are currently taking metformin 500mg three times a day. You do not have any allergies. Your father died of a heart attack aged 50 and your mother also has type 2 diabetes. You have been a cigarette smoker for about 20 years and smoke approximately 20 cigarettes a day. You drink two to three pints of lager a day. You are a heavy goods vehicle driver and therefore do not get much exercise. You admit that your diet is not very good and that you eat a lot of fried foods.

*Your main concern is that the pain is getting worse and you are wondering what the doctor is going to do about the pain.*

# Mark Scheme for Examiner

## Introduction

| | | | | |
|---|---|---|---|---|
| Clean hands, introduce self, confirm patient identity and gain consent for history taking | | | | |

## Limb Pain History

| | | | | | |
|---|---|---|---|---|---|
| Site | | | | | |
| Onset (If pain occurs on exertion what is the claudication distance?) | | | | | |
| Character | | | | | |
| Radiation | | | | | |
| Timing and duration | | | | | |
| Exacerbating factors | | | | | |
| Relieving factors | | | | | |
| Severity | | | | | |
| Previous episodes of limb pain | | | | | |

## Associated Symptoms

| | | | | | |
|---|---|---|---|---|---|
| Foot ulcers | | | | | |
| Sensory changes | | | | | |
| Feeling of reduced temperature in the lower limbs | | | | | |
| Muscle weakness | | | | | |
| Impotence | | | | | |
| Angina | | | | | |

## Past History

| | | | | | |
|---|---|---|---|---|---|
| Atrial fibrillation | | | | | |
| Ischaemic heart disease, stroke, peripheral vascular disease | | | | | |
| Diabetes mellitus | | | | | |
| Hypertension | | | | | |
| High cholesterol | | | | | |
| Past surgical history (including angioplasty, bypass) | | | | | |

## Drug History

| | | | | | |
|---|---|---|---|---|---|
| Drug history | | | | | |
| Allergy history | | | | | |

## Family History

| | | | | | |
|---|---|---|---|---|---|
| Family history | | | | | |

## Social History

| | | | | | |
|---|---|---|---|---|---|
| Smoking status. Duration and quantity of cigarettes smoked | | | | | |
| Alcohol history | | | | | |
| Lifestyle (diet, exercise) | | | | | |
| Occupation | | | | | |

## Finishing the Consultation

| | | | | | |
|---|---|---|---|---|---|
| Elicit patient concerns | | | | | |
| Summarise history back to patient | | | | | |
| Thank patient and close consultation | | | | | |

## General Points

| | | | | |
|---|---|---|---|---|
| Polite to patient | | | | |
| Maintain good eye contact | | | | |
| Appropriate use of open and closed questions | | | | |
| Presentation of case | | | | |

## Questions And Answers for Candidate

### What are the P's associated with acute arterial occlusion of the limb?

- Pain, pallor, pulseless, parasthesia, paralysis and a perishingly cold limb

### What is Buerger's angle?

- Buerger's angle (or the vascular angle) is the angle to which the leg must be raised before it (and the foot) becomes pale. In a normal circulation the toes should remain pink even up to 90 degrees.

**How would you locate the femoral artery clinically in the absence of a pulsation (i.e. due to acute embolism)?**

- The femoral artery is located at the mid-inguinal point. This landmark is half way between the anterior superior iliac spine and the pubic symphysis. The surgeon may use their landmark to plan their embolectomy. Equally this knowledge could be used during a cardiac arrest to obtain an ABG sample.

## Additional Questions to Consider

1 // What signs on examination would suggest chronic arterial insufficiency?

2 // How do you treat acute arterial embolism of the lower limb, for example in the femoral artery?

3 // What diseases are strongly associated with the development of intermittent claudication?

4 // What is the underlying pathophysiology that leads to arterial insufficiency?

5 // What are the differences between an arterial ulcer, a venous ulcer and a neuropathic ulcer of the leg?

6 // What is the name of the malignant transformation that may occur in chronic ulceration?

# Station 7
# BACK PAIN HISTORY

**Candidate Briefing:** Mrs. Fletcher is a 60-year-old lady who is suffering from back pain. She has also become incontinent and is feeling unsteady on her feet. Please take a history and present your findings.

**Patient Briefing:** You are 60 years old and you are called Mrs. Fletcher. You have presented to the emergency department because you have been suffering from back pain. You have also become incontinent and are feeling unsteady on your feet.

You report that the pain is in your lower back. The pain has been gradually worsening over the past two days, however today you have also become incontinent and unsteady on your feet. The pain is relatively sharp and radiates down the back of both legs. The pain is mostly constant and is present at night time. The pain is made worse by movement and is slightly better if you stay still. The pain is currently 9/10 in severity. You have not had any history of trauma or back pain in the past.

You have noticed over the course of today that you have had difficulty with walking and you feel that your legs have become weak. You have also felt some numbness when you wipe you bottom after opening your bowels (you cannot feel the paper against your bottom). You have been finding it difficult to control your bladder and bowel motions, something which is new for you. You have not had any fevers or night sweats. You have lost about 2 stone in the last 6 weeks and have not been trying to lose weight.

You were diagnosed with breast cancer recently although you have been waiting for a staging CT scan to see if the breast cancer had spread anywhere else. You do not take any medications and you do not have any drug allergies. Your mother also had breast cancer aged 50 years old. You are an ex-smoker, having quit 10 years ago. You used to smoke 20 cigarettes a day for 30 years. You do not drink alcohol and you are a retired shop owner.

*Your main concern is that you have been unable to control your bladder and bowel motions. You are hoping that the doctor will be arranging some tests to determine what is causing your back pain.*

## Mark Scheme for Examiner

## Introduction

| | | | | |
|---|---|---|---|---|
| Clean hands, introduce self, confirm patient identity and gain consent for history taking | | | | |

## Back Pain History

| | | | | |
|---|---|---|---|---|
| Site | | | | |
| Onset | | | | |
| Character | | | | |
| Radiation | | | | |
| Timing and duration | | | | |
| Exacerbating factors | | | | |
| Relieving factors | | | | |
| Severity | | | | |
| History of trauma | | | | |
| Previous episodes of back pain | | | | |

## Associated Symptoms

| | | | | |
|---|---|---|---|---|
| Gait disturbance | | | | |
| Weakness | | | | |
| Altered sensation (including saddle anesthesia) | | | | |
| Disturbance of bladder or bowel control | | | | |
| Fever, night sweats | | | | |
| Weight loss | | | | |

## Past Medical History

Past medical history (specifically ask about malignancy)

## Drug History

Drug and allergy history

## Family History

Family history

## Social History

Smoking and alcohol history

Occupation

## Finishing the Consultation

Elicit patient concerns

Summarise history back to patient

Thank patient and close consultation

## General Points

Polite to patient

Maintain good eye contact

Appropriate use of open and closed questions

Presentation of case

The Unofficial Guide to Passing OSCEs: *Candidate Briefings, Patient Briefings and Mark Schemes*

# Questions And Answers for Candidate

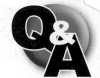

## Define the term "pathological fracture".

- A pathological fracture is one which occurs in diseased bone. Typically this is often due to a metastatic deposit, however it also includes osteoporosis, metabolic bone disorders, inherited disorders, infected bone and cysts.

## List some risk factors for osteoporosis.

- The risk factors for the development of osteoporosis could be classified into those which are modifiable and those which are not
- Among the non-modifiable I would include advancing age, female sex, oestrogen deficiency (e.g. menopause) and a family history
- The modifiable risks include alcohol, smoking, vitamin D deficiency, steroid excess (both endogenous and exogenous), malnutrition, renal disease and physical inactivity

## What is Paget's disease of the bone?

- Paget's disease of the bone is a disease of abnormal bone turnover and remodeling. It is a chronic disorder that weakens bones over time resulting in pain, misshapen bones, and fractures of these bones. Unlike osteoporosis, Paget's disease is localized, usually affecting one or a few bones.

1 // If there are no worrying features on history or examination, and you suspect mechanical causes, how would you treat this?

2 // What is "sciatica"?

3 // What is ankylosing spondylitis? What is the male-female preponderance? List some of the radiological changes seen on a spinal radiograph.

4 // What bones are classically at risk of fracture in osteoporosis?

5 // What is multiple myeloma?

6 // List some common side effects of the medications used to treat mechanical back pain.

# Station 8
# HAEMATOLOGICAL HISTORY

*Candidate Briefing: Mrs. Bee is a 44-year-old lady who reports feeling increasingly tired over the last few weeks. She has lost a considerable amount of weight and also reports increased sweating. Her partner notes that she appears more pale than usual. Please take a history from Mrs. Bee and present your findings.*

*Patient Briefing: You are a 44 year old lady and your name is Mrs. Bee. You have presented to the clinic feeling increasingly tired and unwell over the last few weeks. Your partner has also noted that you appear more pale than usual.*

You report that you have been feeling generally unwell and hot a lot of the time. You have had night sweats five times in the last two weeks and each time you have had to change your clothes and the bed sheets because they are so wet. You have also lost 8kg in the last 3 months even though you have not been trying to lose weight. You have occasionally been feeling light-headed and also short of breath when you climb the stairs, but not at rest. You have not had any palpitations or chest pain.

You have not had any general bleeding, nose bleeds, gum bleeding or blood blisters. You have not coughed up any blood or noticed any in your urine and your periods have not been excessively heavy. You have not noticed that you bleed for longer after trauma and have not had any operations recently. You have not experienced any problems with increased bruising.

If questioned you admit that you have noticed some swellings in your neck and under both of your arm pits. You noticed them a couple of weeks ago and they appear to have been enlarging although they are not tender.

Prior to all of these symptoms you were previously fit and well with no medical conditions. You have never had cancer in the past and have not had any problems with recurrent infections. You do not take any regular medications and you do not have any drug allergies. There is no significant family history. You are a non-smoker. You drink about 2-4 glasses of wine 3-4 evenings a week. You are a typist and have not been exposed to any pesticides or other harmful agents during your work. You have not had any recent travel or contact with anyone else that has been unwell.

*Your main concern is that you are no longer able to do your job due to your symptoms and you are hoping to have some tests to find out what is wrong with you.*

## Mark Scheme for Examiner

## Introduction

Clean hands, introduce self, confirm patient identity and gain consent for history taking

## Symptoms of Anaemia

Tiredness, light headedness, shortness of breath, palpitations, chest pain

## Sweating

Duration

Timing (e.g. at night)

Quantity (i.e. do they need to change bed clothes?)

## Weight loss

Quantify amount of weight lost, and determine if intentional

## Bleeding

Epistaxis

Gum bleeding

Blood blisters

Haemoptysis, haematuria

Menorrhagia (if appropriate)

Prolonged bleeding after surgery or trauma

The Unofficial Guide to Passing OSCEs: *Candidate Briefings, Patient Briefings and Mark Schemes*

## Bruising

| Site | | | | | |
|---|---|---|---|---|---|
| Amount | | | | | |
| Petechiae, purpura, ecchymosis | | | | | |
| Precipitating causes | | | | | |

## Noticeable Lumps (e.g. enlarged lymph nodes)

| Location, duration, tenderness | | | | | |
|---|---|---|---|---|---|

## Past Medical History

| Past medical history (including malignancy, and infections) | | | | | |
|---|---|---|---|---|---|

## Drug History

| Drug and allergy history | | | | | |
|---|---|---|---|---|---|

## Family History

| Family history | | | | | |
|---|---|---|---|---|---|

## Social History

| Smoking and alcohol history | | | | | |
|---|---|---|---|---|---|
| Occupation and exposure to carcinogens (e.g. pesticides) | | | | | |
| Recent travel and infective contacts | | | | | |

## Finishing the Consultation

| Elicit patient concerns | | | | | |
|---|---|---|---|---|---|
| Summarise history back to patient | | | | | |
| Thank patient and close consultation | | | | | |

## General Points

| | | | | | |
|---|---|---|---|---|---|
| Polite to patient | | | | | |
| Maintain good eye contact | | | | | |
| Appropriate use of open and closed questions | | | | | |
| Presentation of case | | | | | |

## Questions And Answers for Candidate

### Broadly classify the causes of anaemia.

- Increased blood loss or red-cell breakdown, defective (dietary) or inadequate (marrow failure) production of red blood cells. It is also acceptable to classify an anaemia histologically in terms of the mean corpuscular volume (MCV) – low MCV, high MCV and normal MCV.

### What is the name of the pathognomic cell that is seen on microscopy in Hodgkin's Disease?

- The Reed-Sternberg cell, which is a giant cell, and visible on microscopy

## List some common causes of an iron deficiency anaemia.

- The common causes stem from GI blood loss and would include peptic ulceration, cancer anywhere in the GI tract, drugs such as aspirin, NSAIDs or anticoagulants, and hereditary diseases such as angiodysplasia and hereditary haemorrhagic telangectasia

## Additional Questions to Consider

1 // What do you understand by the terms lymphoproliferative disorder and myeloproliferative disorder?

2 // What are hypersegmented neutrophils? What conditions might they occur in?

3 // What is the difference between a leukaemia and a lymphoma?

4 // What is the difference between an acute leukaemia and a chronic leukaemia? What age groups do they affect?

5 // How are the lymphomas broadly classified?

6 // How would you investigate a microcytic anaemia?

7 // How would you investigate a macrocytic anaemia?

# Station 9
# BREAST HISTORY

**Candidate Briefing: Mrs. Patterson is a 45-year-old lady who has noticed a lump in her left breast. Please take a history considering her risk factors for breast cancer and present your findings.**

**Patient Briefing: You are a 45-year-old lady and your name is Mrs. Patterson. You have attended the clinic because you have noticed a lump in your left breast.**

You noticed a lump in your left breast about 3 months ago and since then it appears to have increased in size but not changed consistency. The lump is not painful and there was no preceding trauma. Your nipple has not changed in appearance but you have had some blood stained discharge. You aren't sure if you have noticed changes in the lump in relation to your menstrual cycle. You certainly haven't had any breast lumps in the past and you are not breastfeeding at the moment.

You have not noticed any swellings in your arm pits or anywhere else. You have lost about a stone in weight over the last month which is not intentional. You are not short of breath and have not had any back ache.

You have never taken the oral contraceptive pill or used hormone replacement therapy. You have not had breast cancer in the past. You have smoked about 20 cigarettes a day for the last 40 years. You started having periods when you were 15 years old and you believe you are going through the menopause at the moment. You have not had any children. Your sister had breast cancer aged 50 years old.

You do not have any significant medical history. You do not take any medications and have no allergies. Apart from your sister having breast cancer there is no other family history of note. You drink 1-2 glasses of wine a night and work as a secondary school teacher.

**Your main concern is that you have breast cancer and you are hoping to find out what tests the doctor is going to do for this breast lump.**

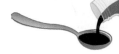

## Mark Scheme for Examiner

## Introduction

| Clean hands, introduce self, confirm patient identity and gain consent for history taking | | | | | |
|---|---|---|---|---|---|

## Breast Lump History

| | | | | | |
|---|---|---|---|---|---|
| Site | | | | | |
| Duration | | | | | |
| Change in size / consistency | | | | | |
| Pain | | | | | |
| Preceding trauma | | | | | |
| Breast or nipple changes | | | | | |
| Nipple discharge | | | | | |
| Changes in relation to menstrual cycle | | | | | |
| Previous breast lumps | | | | | |
| Breastfeeding | | | | | |

## Associated Symptoms

| | | | | | |
|---|---|---|---|---|---|
| Other lumps or swellings | | | | | |
| Weight loss | | | | | |
| Shortness of breath | | | | | |
| Backache | | | | | |

## Risk Factors for Breast Cancer

| | | | | | |
|---|---|---|---|---|---|
| Oral contraceptive pill use | | | | | |
| Hormone replacement therapy use | | | | | |
| Previous breast cancer | | | | | |
| Smoking | | | | | |
| Age of menarche | | | | | |
| Age of menopause | | | | | |
| Previous pregnancy | | | | | |
| Family history of breast cancer | | | | | |

## Past Medical History

| | | | | | |
|---|---|---|---|---|---|
| Past medical history | | | | | |

## Drug History

| | | | | | |
|---|---|---|---|---|---|
| Drug and allergy history | | | | | |

## Family History

| | | | | | |
|---|---|---|---|---|---|
| Family history | | | | | |

## Social History

| | | | | | |
|---|---|---|---|---|---|
| Alcohol intake | | | | | |
| Occupation | | | | | |

## Finishing the Consultation

| | | | | | |
|---|---|---|---|---|---|
| Elicit patient concerns | | | | | |
| Summarise history back to patient | | | | | |
| Thank patient and close consultation | | | | | |

The Unofficial Guide to Passing OSCEs: *Candidate Briefings, Patient Briefings and Mark Schemes*

## General Points

| | | | | | |
|---|---|---|---|---|---|
| Polite to patient | | | | | |
| Maintain good eye contact | | | | | |
| Appropriate use of open and closed questions | | | | | |
| Presentation of case | | | | | |

## Questions And Answers for Candidate

### What is the lymphatic drainage of the breast?

- 75% of the drainage is via the ipsilateral axillary lymph nodes, the remainder is via the parasternal nodes, the other breast or abdominal lymphatics

### What ways might breast cancer be classified?

It can be classified in terms of:
- histopathology (lobular or ductal carcinoma)
- grade (degree of differentiation of the cancerous cell compared to normal breast tissue)
- stage (often TMN – this includes the cancers-in-situ)
- receptor status e.g. oestrogen (ER) progestogen receptor (PR) HER2 (Human Epidermal growth factor Receptor 2)
- DNA assays

## What is a sentinel node biopsy?

- The sentinel node is hypothetically the first node (or group of nodes) that a cancer would drain to and thus metastasise. Therefore, the sentinel node(s) may be free of cancer due to the primary tumour being detected sufficiently early enough.

## Additional Questions to Consider

**1 //** List some of the worrying symptoms in a breast history that would raise your suspicion for underlying cancer?

**2 //** What features on clinical examination would worry you?

**3 //** What features in a history of mastalgia might reassure you that the cause was not sinister?

**4 //** What is a radical mastectomy?

**5 //** What is the name given to the ligaments that support the breast and maintain structural integrity?

**6 //** What are the causes of mastitis?

**7 //** What is the differential diagnosis of a breast lump?

**8 //** What factors might be considered protective against the development of breast cancer?

# Station 10
# SEXUAL HISTORY: VAGINAL DISCHARGE

*Candidate Briefing: Margaret Ford is a 23-year-old woman who has developed vaginal discharge for the last few days. Take a full sexual history and present your findings.*

*Patient Briefing: You are 23 years old and your name is Margaret Ford. You have developed vaginal discharge over the last few days.*

You developed vaginal discharge 3 days ago. The discharge is thick, white, odourless and associated with itching. You have not noticed any new lumps, rashes or ulcers. It is not painful to have intercourse and you have not had any abdominal pain.

You have not noticed any yellow discoloration of your skin. You have not had any eye or joint symptoms, mouth ulcers, fever, lethargy, loss of appetite or weight loss. Your periods are regular. You have not noticed any burning when you pass urine and your bowels are normal. You last had sexual intercourse with a man 5 days ago. He was a one night stand who you had not met before. You had vaginal intercourse with him and did not use a condom as you are currently taking the combined oral contraceptive pill.

Prior to this you have had 9 other sexual partners in the last three months. You only had vaginal intercourse but did not use a condom on any of these occasions. One of the men you had intercourse with was from south-east Asia; otherwise all of the other men were from the UK. You have not travelled abroad recently. You have never paid for sex and never had a same-sex relationship. A number of your previous sexual partners have been bi-sexual. You have never had any testing for sexually transmitted infections, HIV or hepatitis B before and you have never had a blood transfusion. You have 2 tattoos but they were both performed in the UK in a tattoo parlour. You have never injected recreational drugs. You are normally fit and well with no medical problems. You have never had an operation and never been pregnant. Your periods are regular at the moment, you usually have 5 days of bleeding and your last period was 2 weeks ago. You take the combined oral contraceptive pill and no other medications. Only if asked specifically, you have not missed any doses of the contraceptive pill. You do not have any drug allergies. There is no significant family history. You smoke 20 cigarettes a day and have done so for 8 years. You do not drink alcohol in the week but at the weekend can consume up to 20 units in one night. You are currently a student at university.

*Your main concern is that you have picked up a sexually transmitted infection from your most recent sexual partner. You are hoping that the doctor will be able to perform some tests and give you the right treatment.*

# Mark Scheme for Examiner

## Introduction

| | | | | | |
|---|---|---|---|---|---|
| Clean hands, introduce self, confirm patient identity and gain consent for history taking | | | | | |
| Assure patient that all responses are confidential | | | | | |
| Explain that some questions may be sensitive and that you ask all patients the same questions | | | | | |

## Genitourinary Symptoms

| | | | | | |
|---|---|---|---|---|---|
| Discharge (vaginal or urethral) | | | | | |
| Discharge colour and odour | | | | | |
| Noticeable lumps | | | | | |
| Rash | | | | | |
| Ulcers | | | | | |
| Dyspareunia | | | | | |
| Lower abdominal pain | | | | | |

## Systemic Symptoms

| | | | | | |
|---|---|---|---|---|---|
| Jaundice | | | | | |
| Eye symptoms | | | | | |
| Joint symptoms | | | | | |
| Mouth ulceration | | | | | |
| Lethargy, anorexia, weight loss | | | | | |
| Urinary symptoms | | | | | |
| Bowel symptoms | | | | | |

Histories

## Sexual History

| | | | | | |
|---|---|---|---|---|---|
| Last sexual contact, and whether they are a regular partner | | | | | |
| Male or female partner | | | | | |
| Type of sexual contact (oral/vaginal/anal). If male to male sexual contact was it active or passive? | | | | | |
| Condom usage including breakage | | | | | |
| Additional contraception | | | | | |
| Detail other sexual partners in the last 3 months (including type of sexual contact, active or passive sex, and use of barrier protection) | | | | | |
| Foreign travel and sexual partners abroad | | | | | |
| Paying for sex | | | | | |
| Previous same sex relationships | | | | | |
| Previous partners having STIs | | | | | |

## Previous GUM Testing

| | | | | |
|---|---|---|---|---|
| Previous STI, HIV, Hepatitis B check | | | | |
| Previous Hepatitis B vaccination | | | | |

## HIV Risk Factors

| | | | | |
|---|---|---|---|---|
| Receiving blood transfusion (If so, where and when) | | | | |
| Tattoos | | | | |
| Recreational IV drug use | | | | |

## Past Medical History

| | | | | |
|---|---|---|---|---|
| Past medical history | | | | |

Histories

## Obstetric And Gynaecological History

| | | | | | |
|---|---|---|---|---|---|
| Periods (regularity, duration of bleeding, last period) | | | | | |
| Previous pregnancies, miscarriages, abortions | | | | | |
| Use of tampons | | | | | |

## Drug History

| | | | | | |
|---|---|---|---|---|---|
| Drug and allergy history (including recent antibiotics) | | | | | |

## Family History

| | | | | | |
|---|---|---|---|---|---|
| Family history | | | | | |

## Social History

| | | | | | |
|---|---|---|---|---|---|
| Smoking and alcohol history | | | | | |
| Occupation | | | | | |

## Finishing the Consultation

| | | | | | |
|---|---|---|---|---|---|
| Elicit patient concerns | | | | | |
| Summarise history back to patient | | | | | |
| Thank patient and close consultation | | | | | |

## General Points

| | | | | | |
|---|---|---|---|---|---|
| Polite to patient | | | | | |
| Maintain good eye contact | | | | | |
| Asks questions in a sensitive and nonjudgmental manner | | | | | |
| Appropriate use of open and closed questions | | | | | |
| Presentation of case | | | | | |

### How would you manage a possible STD?

Follow the 6 point plan:
- Accurate diagnosis
- Treat symptomatic disease and prevent complications
- Bring back to test for cure
- Contact tracing
- Screen for other STIs
- Council appropriately

### What is bacterial vaginosis?  How is it treated?

- It is an overgrowth or imbalance of normally occurring vaginal flora but is often mistaken for candida infection. Metronidazole or clindamycin are effective treatments, though the condition can recur.

## ? Additional Questions to Consider

1 // Please give some of the common causes of menorrhagia?

2 // List some of the common causes of dysmenorrhea?

3 // What are the short term symptoms reported in chlamydia infection? What are the long term sequelae?

4 // How is chlamydia treated?

5 // What do you understand by the term post-exposure prophylaxis?

6 // Can you name some of the AIDS defining illnesses?

7 // What is toxic shock syndrome and how does it present?

8 // What are the 4 stages of syphilis?

# Chapter 2

# Examination

# Station 1
# CARDIOVASCULAR EXAMINATION

*Candidate Briefing:* **You are the junior doctor on-call, and have been asked to review a 60-year-old patient who has presented to the Emergency Department with shortness of breath and a new murmur. Please examine them. You may assume there is no hepatomegaly, peripheral oedema, or basal lung crackles.**

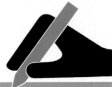

## Mark Scheme for Examiner

### Introduction

| | | | | |
|---|---|---|---|---|
| Clean hands, introduce self, confirm patient identity and gain consent | | | | |
| Patient adequately exposed and positioned comfortably at 45° | | | | |

### General Observation

| | | | | |
|---|---|---|---|---|
| Surroundings (oxygen, monitoring, bedside medication) | | | | |
| Patient (breathlessness, pallor/cyanosis) | | | | |

### Hands

| | | | | |
|---|---|---|---|---|
| Feel for temperature | | | | |
| Look at nails (clubbing, splinter haemorrhages, tar staining, koilonychia) | | | | |
| Look at hands (Osler's nodes, Janeway lesions) | | | | |
| Capillary refill | | | | |

## Pulses

Radial: Rate and rhythm, radio-radial delay

Collapsing pulse

Brachial/carotid (volume and character)

## Face

Eyes (xanthelasma, pallor, corneal arcus)

Cheek (malar flush)

Mouth (central cyanosis)

## JVP

Position the patient – neck turned away, sat at 45°, and look for JVP

Hepatojugular reflux if not seen

## Inspection

Chest wall deformities, visible pulsation, pacemaker/ICD

Scars (median sternotomy, lateral thoracotomy, pacemaker, mitral valvotomy, chest drains)

## Palpation

Apex beat, heaves and thrills

## Auscultation

All four areas of the precordium

Patient rolled to left, holding expiration (mitral stenosis)

Radiation (to axilla and carotids)

| Patient sat up, holding expiration – listen at left sternal edge (aortic regurgitation) | | | | | |
|---|---|---|---|---|---|
| Lung bases | | | | | |

## To Finish

| Feel for hepatomegaly, peripheral/pedal oedema, and perform a peripheral vascular examination | | | | | |
|---|---|---|---|---|---|
| Ask to review observation chart. Check blood pressure, perform fundoscopy, dipstick urine, look at an ECG | | | | | |
| Present findings | | | | | |

## General

| Progressed speedily with confidence | | | | | |
|---|---|---|---|---|---|
| Communicates clear instructions to patient | | | | | |
| Minimises pain and makes patient feel at ease | | | | | |

## Questions And Answers for Candidate

### Name three ways the JVP differs from the carotid pulse.

- JVP has two 'waves', carotid has one
- The internal jugular can be occluded, the carotid cannot be
- The JVP falls with gravity, the carotid should not
- The jugular fills from above after being occluded
- The JVP is impalpable, unlike the carotid pulse
- The JVP falls on inspiration, the carotid should not

## Name three clinical signs of left heart failure.

- Signs of increased work of breathing (e.g. intercostal recession)
- Tachypnea
- Basal lung crackles
- Wheeze
- Cyanosis

## How would you manage a patient in left heart failure secondary to aortic stenosis?

- Initial assessment: Resuscitate using an ABCDE approach
- Initial investigations: ABG, bloods, CXR, ECG, bloods (including FBC, U/Es, CRP (if concerned about infection), troponin (if concerned about an MI))
- Initial management: Monitor heart rate, blood pressure, respiratory rate, oxygen saturations, and urine output. Sit patient up, consider loop diuretics, morphine, nitrates, oxygen
- Will require echo for confirmation of aortic stenosis, and consideration of long term management options

1 // What T wave changes are associated with cardiac ischemia?

2 // What clinical features might indicate severe aortic stenosis?

3 // How do you tell the difference between a mitral regurgitation murmur, and an aortic stenosis murmur?

4 // Give two causes of aortic stenosis.

5 // What is the difference in the ECG changes of angina, unstable angina, a non-STEMI and a STEMI?

Examination

# Station 2
# RESPIRATORY EXAMINATION

*Candidate Briefing:* **Please examine this lady's respiratory system, and present your findings.**

## Mark Scheme for Examiner

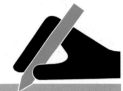

### Introduction

| | | | | | |
|---|---|---|---|---|---|
| Clean hands, introduce self, confirm patient identity and gain consent | | | | | |
| Patient adequately exposed and positioned comfortably at 45° | | | | | |

### General Observation

| | | | | | |
|---|---|---|---|---|---|
| Surroundings (oxygen, monitoring, inhalers, nebulisers, spacers, peak flow meter, sputum pot, chest drains) | | | | | |
| Patient (pallor/cyanosis, cachexia, breathlessness) | | | | | |
| Nature of breathing (hyper/hypoventilation, accessory muscle usage, pursed-lip breathing) | | | | | |
| Added sounds (cough, wheeze, stridor) | | | | | |

### Hands

| | | | | | |
|---|---|---|---|---|---|
| Fingers (clubbing, peripheral cyanosis, tar staining) | | | | | |
| Tremor/$CO_2$ retention flap | | | | | |
| Look at hands (Osler's nodes, Janeway lesions) | | | | | |
| Pulse (rate, rhythm, volume) | | | | | |

## Axilla

Palpate axillary nodes

## Face

Conjunctiva (anaemia)

Horner's syndrome (ptosis, meiosis, enophthalmos, anhydrosis)

Mouth (central cyanosis, candidiasis)

## JVP

Position the patient – neck turned away, sat at 45°, and look for JVP

Hepatojugular reflux if not seen

## Lymph nodes

Neck; from behind. Describe if appropriate

## Inspection of Chest

Patient sitting, fully exposed

Front, axillae and back

Look for lesions on the chest wall (e.g. tumour nodules, neurofibromas), scars (e.g. drains or surgery), and dilated superficial veins

Chest wall movements (intercostal recession, flail chest)

## Palpation

| | | | | | |
|---|---|---|---|---|---|
| Any local abnormalities, trachea (is it central?), apex beat | | | | | |
| Chest expansion (upper, middle, lower zones) | | | | | |
| Tactile vocal fremitus (if not performing whispering pectoriloquy) | | | | | |

## Percussion

| | | | | | |
|---|---|---|---|---|---|
| Comparing the note on both sides, beginning at the lung apices and working downwards | | | | | |
| Map abnormal areas | | | | | |

## Auscultation

| | | | | | |
|---|---|---|---|---|---|
| Ask patient to take deep breaths through an open mouth | | | | | |
| Listen to anterior, lateral, posterior chest wall | | | | | |
| Comparing both sides, alternating left/right, working downwards from above the clavicle to below 11th rib | | | | | |
| Whispering pectoriloquy | | | | | |

## To Finish

| | | | | | |
|---|---|---|---|---|---|
| Review observation chart. Inspect sputum pot | | | | | |
| Assess peak flow | | | | | |
| Present findings | | | | | |

## General

| | | | | | |
|---|---|---|---|---|---|
| Progressed speedily with confidence | | | | | |
| Communicates clear instructions to patient | | | | | |
| Minimises pain and makes patient feel at ease | | | | | |

Examination

## What are three causes of interstitial lung disease?

- Idiopathic
- Extrinsic allergic alveolitis (pigeon fancier's lung, farmer's lung)
- Autoimmune (rheumatoid arthritis, systemic sclerosis, ankylosing spondylitis)
- Occupational (asbestosis, pneumoconiosis, silicosis)
- Drugs (methotrexate, amiodarone, bleomycin, nitrofurantoin)
- Familial

## List four complications of pneumonia.

- (Type 1) Respiratory failure
- Atrial fibrillation
- Pleural effusion
- Empyema
- Lung abscess
- Septicaemia/septic shock
- Pericarditis/myocarditis

## What investigations are available to help support a diagnosis of a pulmonary embolus?

- D-dimer
- Imaging – V/Q scans or CTPA

## Give three causes of a type 2 respiratory failure.

- Any cause of type 1 respiratory failure, if severe enough
- Pulmonary: COPD, asthma, lung fibrosis
- Central decreased respiratory drive: sedatives, CNS tumours, trauma
- Neuromuscular disease: cervical cord lesion, diaphragmatic paralysis, myasthenia gravis and Guillain-Barre syndrome
- Thoracic wall defects: flail chest, kyphoscoliosis

## Additional Questions to Consider

1 // How would you manage a 45 year old male with a CURB score 1 community acquired pneumonia?

2 // Would myasthenia gravis be likely to cause a type 1 or type 2 respiratory failure?

3 // What extrapulmonary features might mycoplasma pneumonia be associated with?

4 // What factors might precipitate an asthma attack?

5 // What type and location of tumour would cause a Horner's syndrome?

# Station 3
# CRANIAL NERVE EXAMINATION

*Candidate Briefing:* **Mr. Wade is a 48 year-old smoker with progressive left-sided neck and arm pain. Please examine this man's cranial nerves and then present your findings.**

## Mark Scheme for Examiner

### Introduction

| | | | | | |
|---|---|---|---|---|---|
| Clean hands, introduce self, confirm patient identity and gain consent | | | | | |

### General Observation

| | | | | | |
|---|---|---|---|---|---|
| Look for ptosis (III), at eye position (III, IV, VI), pupil symmetry (II, III), facial symmetry (VII), sternocleidomastoid/trapezius bulk (XI), listen to speech (V, VII, IX, X, XII) | | | | | |
| Look for exophthalmos/enophthalmos of eye | | | | | |

### CN I (Olfactory)

| | | | | | |
|---|---|---|---|---|---|
| Ask if noticed any changes in smell/taste | | | | | |

### CN II (Optic)

| | | | | | | |
|---|---|---|---|---|---|---|
| Acuity: | Asks if wears glasses<br>One eye at a time with Snellen chart | | | | | |
| Visual fields: | 4 quadrants of eyes, separately<br>Check for neglect by checking both eyes together | | | | | |
| Test blind spot | | | | | | |

## CN III, IV, VI (Oculomotor, trochlear, abducens)

| | | | | | |
|---|---|---|---|---|---|
| Movements (note diplopia, nystagmus, strabismus) | | | | | |
| Accommodation reflex | | | | | |
| Pupillary reflex (direct and consensual) | | | | | |

## CN V (trigeminal)

| | | | | | |
|---|---|---|---|---|---|
| Sensation: Demonstrate centrally on sternum / Each division, each side, with patient's eyes closed / Test light touch, pain, temperature | | | | | |
| Muscles of mastication (temporalis and masseter) – clench, and open jaw | | | | | |
| Offer to test corneal reflex and jaw jerk | | | | | |

## CN VII (facial)

| | | | | | |
|---|---|---|---|---|---|
| Raise eyebrows (temporal branches to facial muscles, differentiate between UMN/LMN lesions) | | | | | |
| Scrunch up eyes (zygomatic) | | | | | |
| Puff out cheeks (buccal) | | | | | |
| Bare teeth, whistle (mandibular) | | | | | |
| Protrude chin (cervical) | | | | | |

## CN VIII (vestibulocochlear)

| | | | | | |
|---|---|---|---|---|---|
| Test hearing whilst occluding contralateral ear; start with 'good' side | | | | | |
| Rinne's test | | | | | |
| Weber's test | | | | | |
| Offer to assess balance | | | | | |

## CN IX, X (glossopharyngeal and vagus)

| | | | | | |
|---|---|---|---|---|---|
| Ask to cough and swallow water | | | | | |
| Patient opens mouth, says 'aah' – check for uvula deviation | | | | | |
| Offer to test gag reflex | | | | | |

## CN XI (accessory)

| | | | | | |
|---|---|---|---|---|---|
| Shrug shoulders against resistance – compare both sides | | | | | |
| Assess sternocleidomastoid against resistance – chin to shoulder | | | | | |

## CN XII (hypoglossal)

| | | | | | |
|---|---|---|---|---|---|
| Inspect tongue for fasciculations whilst inside mouth | | | | | |
| Inspect tongue sticking out for wasting and deviation | | | | | |
| Push tongue against cheek, against examiner resistance | | | | | |

## To Finish

| | | | | | |
|---|---|---|---|---|---|
| Review observation chart | | | | | |
| Offer to formally test smell, perform fundoscopy and to do a peripheral nervous system examination | | | | | |
| Present findings | | | | | |

## General

| | | | | | |
|---|---|---|---|---|---|
| Progressed speedily with confidence | | | | | |
| Communicates clear instructions to patient | | | | | |
| Minimises pain and makes patient feel at ease | | | | | |

## How would you differentiate an upper motor neuron VII lesion from a lower motor neuron VII lesion?

- The forehead muscles have bilateral cortical representation
- In an UMN lesion, there is forehead sparing i.e. the patient would still be able to raise their eyebrows equally on both sides

## What are the characteristics symptoms of a headache due to raised intracranial pressure?

- At their worst first thing in the morning
- Worse on valsalva manoeuvre (coughing, sneezing, straining, bending)
- Associated with other signs of raised intracranial pressure e.g. vomiting (without significant nausea, and early morning), drowsiness, focal neurological signs

## A VIth nerve palsy prevents the eye from doing what movements?

- Abduction of the affected eye

1 // What visual field defect may result from a left occipital lobe lesion?

2 // What visual field defect may result from a right parietal lobe lesion?

3 // A left XIIth nerve palsy will cause the tongue to deviate to the left or the right?

4 // The facial nerve provides taste sensation to which part of the tongue, via which branch?

5 // Define multiple sclerosis

# Station 4: PERIPHERAL NERVE EXAMINATION: UPPER LIMB

*Candidate Briefing:* **Mr. Reilly recently had a fall and fractured his humerus. He is now struggling to perform everyday tasks with his right hand. Please perform a neurological examination of this patient's upper limbs.**

## Mark Scheme for Examiner

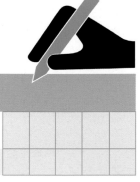

### Introduction

| | | | | | |
|---|---|---|---|---|---|
| Clean hands, introduce self, confirm patient identity and gain consent | | | | | |
| Patient adequately exposed | | | | | |

### General Observation

| | | | | | |
|---|---|---|---|---|---|
| Walking aids, braces, wheelchairs | | | | | |

### Inspection

| | | | | | |
|---|---|---|---|---|---|
| Wasting or hypertrophy, asymmetry, abnormal movements, posture, fasciculations | | | | | |
| Test for pronator drift | | | | | |

### Tone

| | | | | | |
|---|---|---|---|---|---|
| Ensure patient is relaxed and ask about pain | | | | | |
| Passive movements through full range of movement | | | | | |
| Flex elbow | | | | | |
| Supinate forearm | | | | | |
| Circumduct wrist | | | | | |

## Power

| | | | | | |
|---|---|---|---|---|---|
| Patient is given specific instructions, and joints are stabilised during assessment. Movement against resistant, and power reported 0-5 | | | | | |
| Shoulder abduction and adduction | | | | | |
| Elbow flexion and extension (arms out in front) | | | | | |
| Wrist flexion, extension, and circumduction | | | | | |
| Grip strength | | | | | |
| Finger and thumb abduction (fingers spread open) | | | | | |

## Reflexes

| | | | | | |
|---|---|---|---|---|---|
| Biceps | | | | | |
| Brachioradialis | | | | | |
| Triceps | | | | | |
| Use reinforcement if not elicited | | | | | |

## Co-ordination

| | | | | | |
|---|---|---|---|---|---|
| Cerebellar rebound | | | | | |
| Finger-nose test | | | | | |
| Dysdiadokinesia | | | | | |

## Sensation

| | | | | | |
|---|---|---|---|---|---|
| In each dermatome, with patient eyes shut; reference sternum where appropriate | | | | | |
| Light touch | | | | | |
| Pain | | | | | |
| Temperature | | | | | |

| Proprioception | | | | | |
|---|---|---|---|---|---|
| Vibration sense | | | | | |

## To Finish

| Review observation chart; offer to examine the cranial nerves and the lower limbs | | | | | |
|---|---|---|---|---|---|
| Present findings | | | | | |

## General

| Progressed speedily with confidence | | | | | |
|---|---|---|---|---|---|
| Communicates clear instructions to patient | | | | | |
| Minimises pain and makes patient feel at ease | | | | | |

## Questions And Answers for Candidate

### What muscles of the hand are supplied by the median nerve?

- First and second lumbricals

The thenar eminence:
- Opponens pollicis
- Abductor pollicis brevis
- Flexor pollicis brevis

## What are three signs of an ulnar nerve palsy?

- Claw hand
- Weakened little finger abduction
- Weakened 4th and 5th DIP flexion
- Wasting of medial wrist flexors / interossei / medial 2 lumbricals / hypothenar eminence
- Altered sensation over the dorsal and palmar aspects of the medial hand and fingers, up to a vertical line drawn through the ring finger

## Name 3 conditions that may be associated with carpal tunnel syndrome.

- Pregnancy
- Rheumatoid arthritis
- Diabetes mellitus
- Hypothryoidism
- Acromegaly
- Trauma

## Additional Questions to Consider

1 // **What is a common site of trauma to the ulnar nerve?**

2 // **The radial nerve receives nerve fibres from which spinal roots?**

3 // **Wrist drop results from a lesion of which nerve?**

4 // **Vibration sense travels in which spinal tract?**

5 // **Which nerve roots supply the brachioradialis reflex?**

# Station 5: PERIPHERAL NERVE EXAMINATION: LOWER LIMB

*Candidate Briefing:* **Mr. Romberg has long-standing diabetes mellitus. He is concerned that he is continually injuring his feet without realising it. Please perform a neurological examination of this patient's lower limbs.**

## Mark Scheme for Examiner

### Introduction

| | | | | |
|---|---|---|---|---|
| Clean hands, introduce self, confirm patient identity and gain consent | | | | |
| Patient adequately exposed | | | | |

### General Observation

| | | | | |
|---|---|---|---|---|
| Environment: walking aids, braces, wheelchairs, shoes (orthoses) | | | | |

### Inspection

| | | | | |
|---|---|---|---|---|
| Wasting or hypertrophy, asymmetry, abnormal movements, posture, fasciculations | | | | |

### Walking

| | | | | |
|---|---|---|---|---|
| Assess gait | | | | |
| Consider additional tests e.g. tandem walk, Romberg's test if abnormal gait | | | | |

## Tone

| | | | | | |
|---|---|---|---|---|---|
| Lie patient flat on back, ensure relaxed | | | | | |
| Roll legs from side to side, checking resistance of feet | | | | | |
| Lift knee abruptly to check for hypertonia | | | | | |
| Passively flex and extend the knee | | | | | |

## Power

| | | | | | |
|---|---|---|---|---|---|
| Patient is given specific instructions, and joints are stabilised during assessment. Movement against resistance, and power reported 0-5 | | | | | |
| Hip flexion, extension, abduction, adduction | | | | | |
| Knee flexion, extension | | | | | |
| Ankle plantar flexion, dorsiflexion | | | | | |
| Toe flexion, extension | | | | | |

## Reflexes

| | | | | | |
|---|---|---|---|---|---|
| Knee | | | | | |
| Ankle | | | | | |
| Plantar | | | | | |
| Ankle clonus | | | | | |
| Use reinforcement if not elicited | | | | | |

## Co-ordination

| | | | | | |
|---|---|---|---|---|---|
| Heel-shin test | | | | | |
| Finger-nose test | | | | | |
| Dysdiadokinesia | | | | | |

Examination

## Sensation

| | | | | |
|---|---|---|---|---|
| In each dermatome, with patient eyes shut; reference sternum where appropriate | | | | |
| Light touch | | | | |
| Pain | | | | |
| Temperature | | | | |
| Proprioception | | | | |
| Vibration sense | | | | |

## To Finish

| | | | | |
|---|---|---|---|---|
| Review observation chart, offer to examine the cranial nerves, and the upper limbs | | | | |
| Present findings | | | | |

## General

| | | | | |
|---|---|---|---|---|
| Progressed speedily with confidence | | | | |
| Communicates clear instructions to patient | | | | |
| Minimises pain and makes patient feel at ease | | | | |

Examination

## What is Brown-Sequard syndrome? Describe the pattern of sensory loss.

- Results from lateral disruption to one side of the spinal cord
- Ipsilateral loss of dorsal columns:
  Light touch, proprioception, vibration, sense
- Contralateral loss of spinothalamic:
  Pain and temperature

## What signs would be evident in the case of an upper motor neurone lesion compared to a lower motor neurone legion?

- Exaggerated deep tendon reflexes
- Extensor plantar reflex
- Clonus
- Increased tone and spasticity

## Name three symptoms of cauda equina syndrome?

- Back pain radiating down legs
- Decreased sphincter tone
- Bowel and bladder disturbance (typical faecal incontinence, and urinary retention)
- Sensory loss (typically 'saddle anaesthesia')
- Flaccid leg paralysis
- Reduced reflexes in the legs

1 // What nerve roots supply the knee jerk reflex?

2 // Which dermatome covers the majority of the sole of the foot?

3 // What is the usual pattern of sensory loss in diabetic neuropathy?

4 // Which nerve roots contribute to the sciatic nerve?

5 // What are the causes of foot drop?

Examination

# Station 6
## CEREBELLAR EXAMINATION

*Candidate Briefing:* **Mr. Gordon presents to you because of persistent falling whilst walking. He also finds that when reaching for objects, he keeps missing them. Examine his cerebellar function and then present your findings.**

## Mark Scheme for Examiner

### Introduction

| | | | | | |
|---|---|---|---|---|---|
| Clean hands, introduce self, confirm patient identity and gain consent | | | | | |

### General Observation

| | | | | | |
|---|---|---|---|---|---|
| Surroundings (walking aids) | | | | | |
| Patient (dishevelled? Stigmata of liver disease: palmar erythema/spider naevi) | | | | | |

### Gait

| | | | | | |
|---|---|---|---|---|---|
| Normal gait | | | | | |
| Tandem walk | | | | | |

### Eye Signs

| | | | | | |
|---|---|---|---|---|---|
| Slow movements (follow my pen) | | | | | |
| Fast movement (thumb fist test) | | | | | |

## Speech

Listen for slurring speech whilst saying: "british constitution, west register street, baby hippopotamus"

Listen to longer speech for staccato

## Upper Limb

Cerebellar rebound

Finger-nose test

Dysdiadochokinesis

## To Finish

Review observation chart, examine the cranial nerves and peripheral nervous system, perform abdominal examination

Present findings

## General

Progressed speedily with confidence

Communicates clear instructions to patient

Minimises pain and makes patient feel at ease

Examination

---

### What are three causes of a cerebellar syndrome?

- Alcohol
- Drugs e.g. phenytoin
- Multiple sclerosis
- Hereditary ataxias e.g. Friedreich's ataxia
- Tumours of the posterior fossa
- Metastatic disease e.g. from lung or breast
- Infection e.g. varicella zoster or legionella

---

### Describe the gait produced from cerebellar ataxia.

- Feet are separated widely when walking and standing
- Steps are jerky
- Steps vary in size
- The trunk sways
- Gait is impaired especially tandem gait

---

### Occlusion of which arteries may cause a cerebellar stroke syndrome?

- Superior cerebellar artery
- Anterior inferior cerebellar artery
- Posterior inferior cerebellar artery
- Basilar artery

---

1 // Are cerebellar hemisphere signs ipsilateral or contralateral or bilateral?

2 // Is a cerebellar tremor an 'intention' tremor, or a 'resting' tremor?

3 // Would a cerebellar ataxia produce a positive or negative Romberg's test?

4 // What is dysmetria?

5 // What infections might cause a cerebellar syndrome?

Examination

# Station 7
# PARKINSON'S EXAMINATION

*Candidate Briefing:* **Mr. Smith has been referred to your neurology clinic. His GP is concerned that Mr. Smith has signs of Parkinsonism. Please examine the patient for this and present your findings.**

## Mark Scheme for Examiner

### Introduction

| | | | | |
|---|---|---|---|---|
| Clean hands, introduce self, confirm patient identity and gain consent | | | | |

### General Observation

| | | | | |
|---|---|---|---|---|
| Patient in chair, hands on lap | | | | |
| Look for walking aids | | | | |
| Look at face (hypomimia, drooling) | | | | |
| Listen to speech (hypophonia) | | | | |

### Tremor

| | | | | |
|---|---|---|---|---|
| Ask the patient to close eyes and count backwards | | | | |
| Check for postural tremor | | | | |
| Check for intention tremor | | | | |

## Bradykinesia

| | | | | | |
|---|---|---|---|---|---|
| 'Duck's beak' movements | | | | | |
| Piano-playing movements | | | | | |
| Assess writing | | | | | |

## Rigidity

Feel for lead-pipe rigidity
and cogwheeling:    Passively circumduct wrist
Flex / extend elbow
Repeat with other arm

## Gait and Postural Instability

| | | | | | |
|---|---|---|---|---|---|
| Walk normally from one side of the room to the other, turn and come back | | | | | |
| Pull test | | | | | |

## Parkinson-plus Syndromes

| | | | | | |
|---|---|---|---|---|---|
| Eye movements | | | | | |
| Speech | | | | | |
| Hand temperature and capillary refill | | | | | |
| Erect and supine blood pressures | | | | | |

## To Finish

| | | | | | |
|---|---|---|---|---|---|
| Review observation chart. Examine the cranial nerves, and peripheral nervous system | | | | | |
| Present findings | | | | | |

Examination

## General

| | | | | |
|---|---|---|---|---|
| Progressed speedily with confidence | | | | |
| Communicates clear instructions to patient | | | | |
| Minimises pain and makes patient feel at ease | | | | |

## Questions And Answers for Candidate

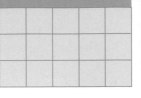

### What are three differential diagnoses of idiopathic Parkinson's disease?

- Vascular Parkinson's disease
- Dementia with Lewy bodies
- Anti-dopaminergic drugs e.g. phenothiazines, metoclopramide
- Multiple system atrophy
- Progressive supranuclear palsy
- Corticobasal degeneration
- Wilson's disease
- Dementia pugilistica

### Describe two positive and two negative symptoms of Parkinson's disease.

- Positive: tremor, chorea, athetosis, dystonia, ballismus, myoclonus
- Negative: bradykinesia (producing reduced facial expression, blinking and postural adjustments); postural disturbance e.g. limb flexion, trunk flexion, and failure to correct imbalances (especially whilst turning or if pushed)

## Describe the tremor seen in Parkinson's disease.

- 'Pill-rolling' tremor
- Decreases with movement
- Occurs at rest
- Around 4-7 Hz (slow)
- Tends to be coarse
- Begins in the distal limbs

## Additional Questions to Consider

1 // What is the first line treatment of Parkinson's Disease?

2 // What other type of drug should be given alongside levodopa in order to reduce peripheral side effects?

3 // What histopathological finding is a hallmark of Parkinson's disease?

4 // What is micrographia?

5 // Is Parkinson's disease more common in males or females?

# Station 8
# GASTROINTESTINAL EXAMINATION

*Candidate Briefing:* **Mr. McClintock has been feeling increasingly tired and confused. His wife feels that Mr. McClintock doesn't look like himself anymore. He has been bruising more easily, and has a long history of excessive alcohol consumption. Please perform a gastrointestinal examination on this gentleman.**

## Mark Scheme for Examiner

### Introduction

| | | | | |
|---|---|---|---|---|
| Clean hands, introduce self, confirm patient identity and gain consent | | | | |
| Patient adequately exposed and positioned lying flat | | | | |

### General Observation

| | | | | |
|---|---|---|---|---|
| Surroundings (look for any drains, or medications at bedside) | | | | |

### Inspection

| | | | | |
|---|---|---|---|---|
| Look for wasting, distension, scars, spider naevi, gynaecomastia, bruising, tattoos, peripheral oedema | | | | |

### Hands

| | | | | |
|---|---|---|---|---|
| Nails (leukonychia, koilonychia, clubbing) | | | | |
| Hands (palmar erythema, Dupuytren's contracture) | | | | |
| Assess for liver flap | | | | |
| Pulse and blood pressure | | | | |

## Face

| Eyes (look for jaundice, anaemia, Kayser-Fleischer rings) | | | | | |
|---|---|---|---|---|---|
| Mouth (gingivitis, ulcers, hydration, peri-oral pigmentation, hepatic fetor) | | | | | |

## Neck

| Lymph nodes (Troisier's sign) | | | | | |
|---|---|---|---|---|---|

## Abdominal Inspection

| Ask if any pain | | | | | |
|---|---|---|---|---|---|
| Look for scars (anterior, posterior, flanks), distension, dilated veins, fullness | | | | | |

## Palpation

| Light and then deep, whilst watching the patients face, and bending to the level of the patient | | | | | |
|---|---|---|---|---|---|
| Liver, spleen, kidneys | | | | | |
| Abdominal aortic aneurysm | | | | | |

## Percussion

| All four quadrants | | | | | |
|---|---|---|---|---|---|
| Liver from above and below | | | | | |
| Spleen | | | | | |
| Percussion tenderness | | | | | |
| Shifting dullness | | | | | |

## Auscultation

Bowel sounds over ileo-caecal valve

Bruits (aorta, renal arteries, liver)

## Hernial Orifices

Place finger over hernia orifice, ask patient to cough

## To Finish

Review observation chart. Perform a PR exam, examine the external genitalia, inspect a stool sample, dipstick the urine

Present findings

## General

Progressed speedily with confidence

Communicates clear instructions to patient

Minimises pain and makes patient feel at ease

## Questions And Answers for Candidate

### What are three causes of ascites?

- Hypoalbuminaemia (cirrhosis, protein malnutrition / malabsorption, nephrotic syndrome)
- Portal hypertension
- Chronic liver disease
- Malignancy (metastatic carcinoma, pelvic carcinoma (ovary))
- Infection (spontaneous bacterial peritonitis, peritoneal tuberculosis)

## Give four differentials for right iliac fossa pain.

- Ectopic pregnancy
- Mesenteric adenitis
- Cystitis
- Cholecystitis
- Diverticulitis
- Salpingitis / PID
- Dysmenorrhoea
- Crohn's disease
- Perforated ulcer
- Meckel's diverticulum
- Food poisoning

## Give four causes of upper gastrointestinal bleeding.

- Mallory-Weiss tear
- Oesophagitis
- Oesophageal varices
- Peptic ulcers
- Gastritis
- Duodenitis
- Malignancy
- Drugs e.g. NSAIDs, steroids, anticoagulants, thrombolytics

1 // What is the difference between a sliding and a rolling hiatus hernia?

2 // Is obstructive jaundice conjugated or unconjugated?

3 // What might cause Grey-Turner's sign?

4 // Which blood test is most sensitive and specific in the diagnosis of acute pancreatitis?

5 // Which areas of the gut does Crohn's disease preferentially affect?

# Station 9
# HERNIA EXAMINATION

*Candidate Briefing:* **Mr. Jarral is a 91 year-old gentleman who has presented with abdominal pain and distension. He has also been vomiting and has noticed a lump in the groin. Please examine this gentleman's groin and present your findings.**

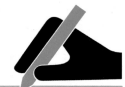

## Mark Scheme for Examiner

### Introduction

| | | | | | |
|---|---|---|---|---|---|
| Clean hands, introduce self, confirm patient identity and gain consent; offer a chaperone | | | | | |
| Adequately expose the patient (umbilicus to knees, with patient standing) | | | | | |

### General Observation

| | | | | | |
|---|---|---|---|---|---|
| Scars, visible masses (pre and post coughing), redness | | | | | |

### Palpation

| | | | | | |
|---|---|---|---|---|---|
| Define local anatomy (pubic tubercle, anterior superior iliac spine, midpoint of the inguinal ligament) | | | | | |
| Feel hernia for tenderness | | | | | |
| Feel for palpable cough impulse | | | | | |
| If patient cannot reduce hernia, attempt to reduce in the Trendelenburg position | | | | | |
| Assess whether the hernia is direct or indirect (is it controlled by pressure over midpoint of inguinal ligament) | | | | | |

## Auscultate

| | | | | | |
|---|---|---|---|---|---|
| Over the hernia | | | | | |

## To Finish

| | | | | | |
|---|---|---|---|---|---|
| Review observation chart | | | | | |
| Examine the contralateral hernia orifice | | | | | |
| Perform an abdominal examination including a PR | | | | | |
| Examine the scrotum | | | | | |
| Present findings | | | | | |

## General

| | | | | | |
|---|---|---|---|---|---|
| Progressed speedily with confidence | | | | | |
| Communicates clear instructions to patient | | | | | |
| Minimises pain and makes patient feel at ease | | | | | |

## Questions And Answers for Candidate

### What are three differentials for a groin lump?

- Hernia
- Lymph node
- Saphena varix
- Abscess
- Undescended testis
- Lipoma

## State two risk factors for inguinal hernias.

- Family history
- Being overweight
- Chronic coughing
- Chronic constipation
- Carrying heavy loads
- Undescended testes or prematurity as an infant

## Additional Questions to Consider

1 // What is the definition of a hernia?

2 // Which is more common, a direct or an indirect hernia?

3 // What is the most serious complication of an inguinal hernia?

4 // Are inguinal hernias more common in males or females?

5 // What structures pass through the femoral canal?

# Station 10
# TESTICULAR EXAMINATION

*Candidate Briefing:* **Mr. Smith is a 20 year-old gentleman who has noticed swelling of his right testicle. Please perform the appropriate examination and present your findings.**

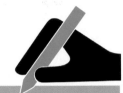

## Mark Scheme for Examiner

### Introduction

| | | | | |
|---|---|---|---|---|
| Clean hands, introduce self, confirm patient identity and gain consent | | | | |
| Ask for a chaperone | | | | |
| Ask the patient to undress from the waist down | | | | |
| Position the patient standing up | | | | |

### Inspection

| | | | | |
|---|---|---|---|---|
| General: Visible pain? Gynaecomastia, secondary sexual characteristics | | | | |
| Scrotum: Size, shape, swelling, asymmetry, ulcers, rashes, scars, pubic hair distribution | | | | |
| Penis: Ulceration and discharge, position of external urethral meatus | | | | |

### Palpation

| | | | | |
|---|---|---|---|---|
| Check if in pain | | | | |
| Size – symmetrical / asymmetrical? Whole testis or discrete mass? | | | | |

| Lumps: | Can you get above it? | | | | | |
|---|---|---|---|---|---|---|
| | Separate from, or part of testis? | | | | | |
| | Cystic or solid? | | | | | |
| | Tender or non-tender? | | | | | |
| | Transilluminate? | | | | | |
| Epididymal head, body, tail | | | | | | |
| Trace spermatic cord | | | | | | |

## To Finish

| | | | | | |
|---|---|---|---|---|---|
| Review observation chart, perform abdominal examination and palpate inguinal nodes, dipstick urine | | | | | |
| Offer to teach testicular self examination | | | | | |
| Present findings | | | | | |

## General

| | | | | | |
|---|---|---|---|---|---|
| Progressed speedily with confidence | | | | | |
| Communicates clear instructions to patient | | | | | |
| Minimises pain and makes patient feel at ease | | | | | |

## Questions And Answers for Candidate

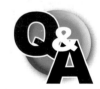

### How would you explain to this patient how to self-examine his testicles in the future?

- Examine whilst in the bath/shower, to soften the skin and make it easier
- Feel for lumps on the skin, and swelling inside the scrotum
- Examine each testicle separately. Then compare the two – remember it can be normal to have one larger and lower
- Use both hands and roll the testicle between the thumb and forefinger
- Seek medical advice if there are any abnormalities or concerns

## Give four differentials for scrotal masses.

- Hydrocoele
- Spermatocoele
- Varicocoele
- Testicular tumour
- Epididymitis
- Orchitis
- Indirect inguinal hernia

## What is the main differential for epididymo-orchitis that must be excluded?

- Testicular torsion

**?**  **Additional Questions to Consider**

1 // What tumour makers may be raised in testicular tumours?

2 // What type of testicular lumps can be transilluminated?

3 // What age group of men commonly get testicular tumours?

4 // What should be the immediate management when testicular torsion is suspected?

5 // Which side do varicoceles classically present on?

# Station 11
# STOMA EXAMINATION

*Candidate Briefing:* **Mr. Pouch has attended a general surgery outpatient clinic. Please examine the stoma bag, and present your findings.**

## Mark Scheme for Examiner

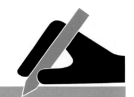

### Introduction

| | | | | | |
|---|---|---|---|---|---|
| Clean hands, introduce self, confirm patient identity and gain consent | | | | | |
| Stoma and surrounding abdomen adequately exposed | | | | | |

### General Observation

| | | | | | |
|---|---|---|---|---|---|
| Signs of infection, fistulae, skin excoriation | | | | | |
| Site (described in relation to abdominal quadrants) | | | | | |
| Bag contents (empty / solid / liquid / urine) | | | | | |
| Surface (flush with skin / protruding spout / single or double lumen / health of mucosa / surrounding skin) | | | | | |
| Abdominal inspection (especially scars to suggest previous surgery) | | | | | |

### Palpation

| | | | | | |
|---|---|---|---|---|---|
| Lubricant to gloved index finger | | | | | |
| Feel for stenosis | | | | | |
| End type – confirm number of openings | | | | | |

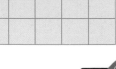

## To Finish

| | | | | | |
|---|---|---|---|---|---|
| Review observation chart; get patient to cough (to exclude parastomal / incisional hernia) | | | | | |
| Replace ostomy appliance | | | | | |
| Perform abdominal and perineal examination | | | | | |
| Present findings | | | | | |

## General

| | | | | | |
|---|---|---|---|---|---|
| Progressed speedily with confidence | | | | | |
| Communicates clear instructions to patient | | | | | |
| Minimises pain and makes patient feel at ease | | | | | |

## Questions And Answers for Candidate

### Name four complications of having a stoma bag?

Immediate:      Haemorrhage

Early:          Ischaemia
                Adhesions
                Diarrhoea

Late:           Skin excoriation
                Parastomal hernia
                Stenosis
                Fistulas
                Psychosexual complications
                Nutrional deficiency
                Prolapse

## What sites should be avoided when choosing where to place a stoma? Give three.

- Near to bony prominences
- Near the umbilicus
- Old wounds and scars
- Skin folds and creases
- The waistline

Examination

## What are three complications of reversing a stoma?

- Ileus
- Small bowel obstruction
- Anastomotic leak
- Fistula formation
- Wound infection
- Hernia

## Additional Questions to Consider

1 // Give two reasons why someone might have an ileostomy.

2 // Why is a spout necessary in an ileostomy? *Protect skin from digestion*

3 // What is a Hartmann's operation and what type of stoma would be created? *end colostomy End colostomy*

4 // What advice would you give to a patient with skin excoriation?

5 // What specific nutrient deficiencies should be watched for in a patient with an ileostomy? *B12*

# Station 12
# RECTAL EXAMINATION

*Candidate Briefing:* **You are a junior doctor seeing an elderly gentleman who has presented with a history of altered bowel habits and PR bleeding. Treat and address the model as you would a real patient and perform a digital rectal examination, stating your positive and negative findings. He has already consented to the procedure.**

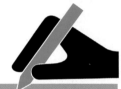

## Mark Scheme for Examiner

### Introduction

| | | | | |
|---|---|---|---|---|
| Clean hands, introduce self, confirm patient identity and gain consent; ask for a chaperone | | | | |
| Ask the patient to undress – removing underwear just before examination | | | | |
| Position in left lateral position | | | | |
| Use incontinence sheet if possible | | | | |
| Wash and glove both hands | | | | |

### Inspection

| | | | | |
|---|---|---|---|---|
| Separate the buttocks | | | | |
| Look for fissures, skin tags, erythema, sinuses / fistulae, pilonoidal sinuses, haemorrhoids | | | | |

## Examination

Lubricate right index finger, insert towards umbilicus

Palpate anterior, right lateral, posterior, left lateral walls

Feel prostate for size, surface, consistency

Comment on presence of masses or stool

Test anal tone

Remove finger, check for blood, mucus, faeces, melaena

Offer tissues, restore dignity

## To Finish

Review observation chart. Perform gastrointestional examination

Present findings

## General

Progressed speedily with confidence

Communicates clear instructions to patient

Minimises pain and makes patient feel at ease

## Name four common causes of rectal bleeding.

- Haemorrhoids
- Anal fissures
- Colon polyps
- Colorectal cancer
- Inflammatory bowel disease (Crohn's disease, ulcerative colitis)
- Intestinal infections
- Diverticular disease
- Angiodysplasia
- Blood loss from upper GI tract (oesophageal varices, gastritis, gastric carcinoma)

## Give two causes or exacerbating factors of haemorrhoids.

- Constipation
- Pelvic tumour
- Pregnancy
- Congestive heart failure
- Portal hypertension

## Give four reasons why a PSA level might be raised.

- Prostatitis
- Urinary tract infection
- Recent ejaculation
- Benign prostatic hyperplasia
- Prostatic carcinoma
- Recent rectal examination

1 // At what points around the anus are haemorrhoids usually located?

2 // Give three causes of melaena

3 // What is the nerve supply of the anal sphincter?

4 // What would the prostate feel like in prostatic carcinoma?

5 // What might cause anal fissures?

Examination

# Station 13
# PERIPHERAL ARTERIAL EXAMINATION

*Candidate Briefing:* **Mr. Smith is a 60-year-old smoker who has developed pain in his right leg on walking. It is present at rest. Please examine the arterial system in his lower limbs and present your findings.**

## Mark Scheme for Examiner

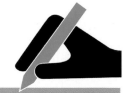

### Introduction

| | | | | |
|---|---|---|---|---|
| Clean hands, introduce self, confirm patient identity and gain consent | | | | |
| Adequately expose patient (remove trousers) | | | | |

### General Observation

| | | | | |
|---|---|---|---|---|
| Look for tar stains, corneal arcus, xanthelasma / xanthoma, surgical scars | | | | |
| Feel pulse | | | | |

### Leg Inspection

| | | | | |
|---|---|---|---|---|
| Scars, skin changes (thickening, thinning, dry), swelling, nail changes, varicose veins, chronic venous disease | | | | |
| Ulcers: Site, shape, depth, edge, quality of base | | | | |
| Looking underneath any dressing | | | | |

## Palpate

| | | | | | |
|---|---|---|---|---|---|
| Temperature | | | | | |
| Capillary refill | | | | | |
| Oedema | | | | | |
| Sensation | | | | | |
| Squeeze calf | | | | | |
| Pulses – use a Doppler if impalpable (femoral, popliteal, dorsalis pedis, posterior tibial) | | | | | |
| Abdominal aorta | | | | | |

## Auscultate

| | | | | | |
|---|---|---|---|---|---|
| Femoral bruits | | | | | |

## Special Tests

| | | | | | |
|---|---|---|---|---|---|
| Perform Buerger's test | | | | | |

## To Finish

| | | | | | |
|---|---|---|---|---|---|
| Review observation chart, measure ABPI, perform fundoscopy | | | | | |
| Dip urine for glucose, protein, blood | | | | | |
| Assess function ability in corridor walking test | | | | | |
| Present findings | | | | | |

## General

| | | | | | |
|---|---|---|---|---|---|
| Progressed speedily with confidence | | | | | |
| Communicates clear instructions to patient | | | | | |
| Minimises pain and makes patient feel at ease | | | | | |

Examination

## What is the anatomical landmark for palpating the posterior tibial pulse?

- Posterior to the medial malleolus

## What comprises 'best medical therapy' for peripheral arterial disease? State three elements.

- Smoking cessation, exercise, weight control
- Antiplatelet agents: aspirin or clopidogrel
- Lipid-lowering agent: usually a statin
- Blood pressure control
- Diabetes control

## What should the ABPI be in a healthy individual?

- Above 0.9

1 // If you were concerned about peripheral arterial disease, what imaging tests might be helpful?

2 // What should the capillary refill time be in a healthy person, and how do you carry out this test?

3 // Which is more painful, an arterial ulcer or a venous ulcer?

4 // What value of ABPI would be consistent with critical limb ischaemia?

Examination

# Station 14
## VARICOSE VEINS

*Candidate Briefing:* **Mr. Wilson is known to suffer from varicose veins. Please examine his legs, and describe any changes that may be associated with venous disease.**

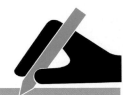

## Mark Scheme for Examiner

### Introduction

| | | | | |
|---|---|---|---|---|
| Clean hands, introduce self, confirm patient identity and gain consent | | | | |
| Adequately expose patient (remove trousers) | | | | |

### Inspection

| | | | | |
|---|---|---|---|---|
| Follow the path of the long saphenous vein | | | | |
| Follow the path of the short saphenous vein | | | | |
| Look for any thread veins | | | | |
| Look for signs of chronic venous disease (lipodermatosclerosis, saphena varix, venous eczema, venous / malleolar flare, skin pigmentation, atrophie blanche, oedema, 'inverted champagne bottle' appearance, venous ulcers) | | | | |

### Palpation

| | | | | |
|---|---|---|---|---|
| Temperature, tendernesss, phlebitis, pitting oedema | | | | |
| Lipodermatosclerosis | | | | |
| Feel for saphenofemoral junction and sapheno-popliteal junction (whilst patient coughs) | | | | |

The Unofficial Guide to Passing OSCEs: *Candidate Briefings, Patient Briefings and Mark Schemes*

## Percussion

Tap test

## Special Test

Trendelenburg test

## To Finish

Review observation chart, perform abdominal examination

Present findings

## General

Progressed speedily with confidence

Communicates clear instructions to patient

Minimises pain and makes patient feel at ease

## Questions And Answers for Candidate

### What are the management options for varicose veins?

Lifestyle changes:     Weight loss and exercise
Education:     Keep the leg elevated, prevent injury, good skin care

- Graded compression stockings
- Surgery if phlebitis, ulcers, bleeding, eczema
- Venous 'stripping' and ligation
- Endovenous procedures e.g. radio frequency or laser ablation of the long or short saphenous vein

## Name three complications of varicose veins.

- Leg ulcers
- Haemorrhage
- Thrombophlebitis
- DVT
- Skin changes

## State three risk factors for varicose veins.

- Increased age
- Being female
- Prolonged standing
- Pregnancy
- Obesity
- Family history

## ? Additional Questions to Consider

1 // What defect in veins causes them to become varicose?

2 // What investigations may be done in a patient with varicose veins?

3 // What are spider veins?

4 // Where on the lower limb are varicose veins commonly found?

5 // What is a saphena varix?

# Station 15
# ULCER EXAMINATION

*Candidate Briefing:* **Mr. Smith is a 67 year-old diabetic. His wife has noticed an ulcer on Mr. Smith's left foot. Please examine this gentleman's skin and present your findings.**

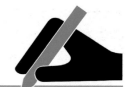

## Mark Scheme for Examiner

### Introduction

| | | | | |
|---|---|---|---|---|
| Clean hands, introduce self, confirm patient identity and gain consent | | | | |

### General Inspection

| | | | | |
|---|---|---|---|---|
| Adequately exposed | | | | |
| Look from all aspects | | | | |
| Site, size, shape, skin, scars, colour, base, edge, depth | | | | |

### Palpation

| | | | | |
|---|---|---|---|---|
| Check pain | | | | |
| Tenderness, temperature, lymph nodes, local tissue | | | | |

## To Finish

| | | | | |
|---|---|---|---|---|
| Review observation chart, measure ABPI | | | | |
| Vascular examination; include pulses, inspection for signs of chronic venous insufficiency | | | | |
| Peripheral neurological examination | | | | |
| Present findings | | | | |

## General

| | | | | |
|---|---|---|---|---|
| Progressed speedily with confidence | | | | |
| Communicates clear instructions to patient | | | | |
| Minimises pain and makes patient feel at ease | | | | |

## Questions And Answers for Candidate

### What are three causes of leg ulcers?

| | |
|---|---|
| Neuropathic: | Often idiopathic |
| | Diabetes mellitus |
| | Alcohol |
| | Vitamin deficiency |
| | |
| Venous: | Varicose veins |
| | Deep vein thrombosis |
| | Immobility of the limb |
| | |
| Arterial: | Atherosclerosis |
| | Diabetes mellitus |
| | Vasculitides |
| | Rheumatoid arthritis |

**What areas are common sites on the foot for neuropathic ulcers? Give three.**

- Malleoli
- Heel
- Metatarsal heads
- 5th metatarsal base

**What is the difference between wet and dry gangrene?**

- Wet gangrene tends to develop much more rapidly
- Wet gangrene is associated with infection
- Dry gangrene is associated with ischaemia
- Dry gangrene usually involves no fluid or pus
- In dry gangrene the appendage often looks black, in wet gangrene it will likely be red
- Wet gangrene is more commonly associated with a foul odour

## Additional Questions to Consider

1 // How would you manage an arterial ulcer?

2 // How would you manage a venous ulcer?

3 // What skin changes might be associated with a venous ulcer?

4 // Give three causes of an arterial ulcer.

5 // What is lipodermatosclerosis?

# Station 16
# NECK LUMP EXAMINATION

*Candidate Briefing:* **Mr. Gardner has been complaining of a lump in his neck. Please examine him and present your findings with a differential diagnosis.**

## Mark Scheme for Examiner

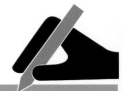

### Introduction

| | | | | |
|---|---|---|---|---|
| Clean hands, introduce self, confirm patient identity and gain consent | | | | |
| Neck adequately exposed | | | | |

### Inspection

| | | | | |
|---|---|---|---|---|
| At eye level | | | | |
| Look at front, sides, back of neck for masses | | | | |
| Describe the mass (site, size, shape, colour, edge, skin) | | | | |
| Ask the patient to open their mouth (look for thyroglossal cyst) | | | | |
| Ask the patient to swallow some water / protrude their tongue (look for movement suggestive of thyroid mass) | | | | |

### Palpation

| | | | | |
|---|---|---|---|---|
| Submandibular, pre / post auricular nodes | | | | |
| Thyroid area whilst the patient swallows / protrudes tongue | | | | |
| Anterior/posterior cervical nodes | | | | |
| Supraclavicular nodes | | | | |

| Parotid nodes | | | | | |
|---|---|---|---|---|---|
| Mastoid nodes | | | | | |
| Occipital nodes | | | | | |
| Describe any lump found (tenderness, temperature, consistency, mobility, pulsatility, bruit, transillumination) | | | | | |

## To Finish

| | | | | | |
|---|---|---|---|---|---|
| Review observation chart: look in the mouth, palpate floor of mouth, look in nose and ears, examine face and scalp | | | | | |
| Present findings | | | | | |

## General

| | | | | | |
|---|---|---|---|---|---|
| Progressed speedily with confidence | | | | | |
| Communicates clear instructions to patient | | | | | |
| Minimises pain and makes patient feel at ease | | | | | |

Examination

### Give four causes of an anterior triangle lump?

Submandibular region:   Submandibular stones

Pulsatile:              Carotid aneurysm
                        Tortuous carotid artery
                        Chemodectoma

Non-pulsatile:          Dermoid cyst
                        Thyroid goitre
                        Thyroglossal cyst
                        Branchial cyst

### What are the three main pairs of salivary glands?

- Submandibular
- Sublingual
- Parotid

**What might cause an enlarged Virchow's node? Give two examples.**

- Intra-abdominal malignancy, particularly gastric
- Breast cancer
- Lung cancer
- Lymphoma
- Infections

Examination

## Additional Questions to Consider

1 // What makes up the borders of the anterior triangle?

2 // What makes up the borders of the posterior triangle?

3 // Are sebaceous cysts subcutaneous or intradermal?

4 // The laryngeal nerve is a branch of which cranial nerve?

5 // At what vertebral level does the carotid artery bifurcate?

# Station 17
# BREAST EXAMINATION

*Candidate Briefing:* **Mrs. Dodds is a 25-year-old lady who has noticed a lump in her left breast. Perform a breast examination and present your findings.**

## Mark Scheme for Examiner

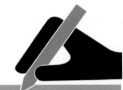

### Introduction

| | | | | |
|---|---|---|---|---|
| Clean hands, introduce self, confirm patient identity and gain consent | | | | |
| Ask for a female chaperone | | | | |
| Ask patient to undress down to waist, sit on edge of the bed | | | | |

### Inspection

| | | | | |
|---|---|---|---|---|
| Inspect in five positions: at rest, arms above head, sitting, pushing up off bed with both hands, hands on hips and pushing inwards, leant forwards | | | | |
| Look for: skin changes (e.g. peau d'orange), nipple changes (e.g. retraction, discharge), general changes (e.g. asymmetry, tethering, lumps) | | | | |

### Palpation

| | | | | |
|---|---|---|---|---|
| Adequately position patient: lying at 45 degrees, arm behind head (on side to be examined); start with normal breast | | | | |
| Report any lumps: size, location, shape, colour, tenderness, temperature, consistency, surface, well / ill-defined, tethering / mobility, overlying skin | | | | |

| All four quadrants with flat of fingers, plus underneath nipple and areola, and axillary tail | | | | | |
|---|---|---|---|---|---|
| Repeat on other breast | | | | | |

## To Finish

| Palpate for hepatomegaly, and bony tenderness, auscultate the lungs | | | | | |
|---|---|---|---|---|---|
| Offer to teach self-examination | | | | | |
| Present findings | | | | | |

## General

| Progressed speedily with confidence | | | | | |
|---|---|---|---|---|---|
| Communicates clear instructions to patient | | | | | |
| Minimises pain and makes patient feel at ease | | | | | |

## Questions And Answers for Candidate

### Name three non malignant causes of breast lumps.

- Fibroadenoma
- Fibrocystic change
- Sebaceous cyst
- Acute mastitis/abscess
- Galactocoele
- Lipoma
- Fat necrosis
- Gynaecomastia

## What does 'triple assessment' in the diagnosis of breast cancer comprise of?

- Clinical examination
- Histology / cytology
- Ultrasonography and / or mammography

## List three risk factors for breast cancer.

- Nulliparity
- First pregnancy over 30 years old
- Early menarche
- Late menopause
- HRT
- Obesity
- BRCA genes
- Family history
- Not breast feeding
- Previous breast cancer

## ? Additional Questions to Consider

1 // For which patients is traztuzumab / Herceptin suitable?

2 // For which patients is tamoxifen suitable?

3 // In what type of breast cancer may Paget's disease of the nipple usually be seen?

4 // What features in a history of mastalgia might reassure you that the cause was not sinister?

5 // What is a radical mastectomy?

# Station 18
# DERMATOLOGY EXAMINATION

*Candidate Briefing:* **Mrs. Barton is a 45 year-old lady who has developed a rash on her scalp and elbows. Please describe the rashes, and come up with a likely list of differentials.**

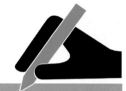

## Mark Scheme for Examiner

### Introduction

| | | | | | |
|---|---|---|---|---|---|
| Clean hands, introduce self, confirm patient identity and gain consent | | | | | |
| Patient adequately exposed | | | | | |

### Characterise the Lesion

| | | | | | |
|---|---|---|---|---|---|
| Describe the shape (round / oval / annular / linear / irregular) | | | | | |
| Describe the outline (well or ill-demarcated) | | | | | |
| Colour | | | | | |
| Smooth or rough surface | | | | | |
| Crust/Scale/Keratin horn/Excoriation/Maceration/Lichenification | | | | | |
| Lift the scale or crust to see what is underneath | | | | | |
| Assess if rash is blanching | | | | | |

## Secondary Sites

| | | | | | |
|---|---|---|---|---|---|
| Nails (psoriasis): Pitting, ridging, discolouration, sub-ungal hyperkeratosis, onycholysis | | | | | |
| Koebner phenomenon (psoriasis) | | | | | |
| Look behind ears and around scalp line (for plaques in psoriasis) | | | | | |
| Fingers and wrists (scabies) | | | | | |
| Toe-webs (fungal) | | | | | |
| Mouth (lichen planus) | | | | | |

## Special Techniques

| | | | | | |
|---|---|---|---|---|---|
| Scrape a psoriatic plaque for capillary bleeding | | | | | |
| Nikolsky's sign | | | | | |

## To Finish

| | | | | | |
|---|---|---|---|---|---|
| Review observation chart | | | | | |
| Present findings | | | | | |

## General

| | | | | | |
|---|---|---|---|---|---|
| Progressed speedily with confidence | | | | | |
| Communicates clear instructions to patient | | | | | |
| Minimises pain and makes patient feel at ease | | | | | |

## Name three nail changes you might you see with psoriasis.

- Pitting
- Ridging
- Discolouration
- Sub-ungal hyperkeratosis
- Onycholysis

## What features may make you suspicious of malignant melanoma?

- Asymmetry
- Borders being irregular
- Colour irregularity
- Diameter over 7mm
- Evolution of the lesion – size and shape
- Symptoms such as itching or bleeding

## What is Köebner phenomenon?

- Skin lesions appearing at the site of trauma e.g. in psoriasis

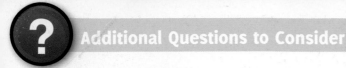

1 // Eczema herpeticum is caused by what?

2 // What pathogen is usually involved in acne vulgaris?

3 // What is Auspitz sign?

4 // What are the possible complications of erythroderma?

5 // Which is more likely to become malignant, squamous cell carcinoma or basal cell carcinoma?

# Station 19
# CUSHING'S EXAMINATION

*Candidate Briefing:* **Mrs. Kain, a 30 year-old lady, presents to your GP surgery with feelings of low mood and having not had a menstrual period for three months. She has also gained weight. She is taking long-term oral steroids for asthma. Please perform a relevant examination of her endocrine system.**

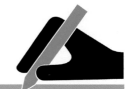

## Mark Scheme for Examiner

### Introduction

| | | | | | |
|---|---|---|---|---|---|
| Clean hands, introduce self, confirm patient identity and gain consent | | | | | |
| Patient adequately exposed | | | | | |

### Hands and Arms

| | | | | | |
|---|---|---|---|---|---|
| Look for bruising especially on the back of hands and forearms | | | | | |
| Look for wounds | | | | | |
| Compare the size of limbs with that of the trunk | | | | | |
| Test skin fold thickness | | | | | |
| Assess for proximal myopathy | | | | | |

### Face

| | | | | | |
|---|---|---|---|---|---|
| Look for mooning, acne, plethoric cheeks, hirsuitism, hair thinning, cataracts | | | | | |

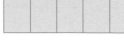

## Neck

| Inspect and feel for fat pads in the supraclavicular fossae | | | | | |
|---|---|---|---|---|---|

## Back

| Inspect and feel for interscapular fat pads | | | | | |
|---|---|---|---|---|---|
| Kyphosis, scoliosis | | | | | |
| Stature | | | | | |
| Loss of distance between lower ribs and top of pelvis | | | | | |

## Chest

| Inspect for breathlessness | | | | | |
|---|---|---|---|---|---|
| Auscultate for wheeze | | | | | |
| Inspect for gynaecomastia | | | | | |

## Abdomen

| Centripetal adiposity | | | | | |
|---|---|---|---|---|---|
| Scars from adrenalectomy | | | | | |
| Striae | | | | | |

## Legs

| Look for thin legs, thin skin, bruises, ulcers, oedema, muscle wasting | | | | | |
|---|---|---|---|---|---|
| Test for proximal myopathy | | | | | |

## To Finish

| Review observation chart including BP | | | | | |
|---|---|---|---|---|---|
| Present findings | | | | | |

## General

| | | | | | |
|---|---|---|---|---|---|
| Progressed speedily with confidence | | | | | |
| Communicates clear instructions to patient | | | | | |
| Minimises pain and makes patient feel at ease | | | | | |

## Questions And Answers for Candidate

### What are three complications of transphenoidal hypophysectomy (treatment for pituitary adenoma)?

- CSF rhinorrhoea
- Diabetes insipidus
- Visual field disturbance
- Persistence of disease
- Recurrence of disease

### Give three causes of a Cushing's syndrome.

- Pituitary adenoma
- Small cell lung cancer
- Carcinoid tumour
- Exogenous steroids
- Adrenal hyperplasia / adenoma / carcinoma

> **What type of visual field defect would arise from an enlarged pituitary gland?**

- Bitemporal hemianopia

## Additional Questions to Consider

1 // What test is done to confirm a diagnosis of Cushing's syndrome?

2 // What might give you a pseudo-Cushing's syndrome?

3 // What skin changes are associated with Cushing's syndrome?

4 // Where are glucocorticosteroids produced in the body?

5 // What is the pattern of obesity seen in Cushing's syndrome?

# Station 20
# ACROMEGALY EXAMINATION

*Candidate Briefing:* **Mr. Black, a 34 year-old man, presents to your GP surgery after noticing his hands and feet have 'swollen up' over the last few months; his wedding ring no longer fits his finger and his shoe size has increased. He also reports increased sweating. Please perform a relevant examination of his endocrine system.**

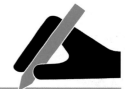

## Mark Scheme for Examiner

### Introduction

| | | | | | |
|---|---|---|---|---|---|
| Clean hands, introduce self, confirm patient identity and gain consent | | | | | |
| Patient adequately exposed | | | | | |

### Hands

| | | | | | |
|---|---|---|---|---|---|
| Size and shape | | | | | |
| Palpate for moistness / bogginess / texture | | | | | |
| Pinch skin on backs of hands for thickness | | | | | |
| Check sensation in the median nerve distribution | | | | | |
| Phalen's test | | | | | |
| Tinel's test | | | | | |
| Radial pulse | | | | | |

## Arms

| | | | | | |
|---|---|---|---|---|---|
| Check for axillary hair loss | | | | | |
| Proximal myopathy | | | | | |

## Face

| | | | | | |
|---|---|---|---|---|---|
| Inspect for prominent supra-orbital ridges, prognathism, large nose / ears / lips / tongue, coarse facial appearance | | | | | |
| Ask patient to stick out tongue – check size | | | | | |
| Look at gums for diastema | | | | | |
| Check for husky voice | | | | | |
| Assess visual fields | | | | | |

## Neck

| | | | | | |
|---|---|---|---|---|---|
| Check JVP | | | | | |
| Feel for goitre | | | | | |

## Chest

| | | | | | |
|---|---|---|---|---|---|
| Feel for apex beat | | | | | |
| Auscultate the precordium for a third heart sound | | | | | |
| Auscultate the lung bases | | | | | |

## Abdomen

| | | | | | |
|---|---|---|---|---|---|
| Assess for hepatomegaly | | | | | |

The Unofficial Guide to Passing OSCEs: *Candidate Briefings, Patient Briefings and Mark Schemes*

## Legs

| | | | | |
|---|---|---|---|---|
| Proximal myopathy | | | | |
| Look for enlarged feet | | | | |
| Check heel pad thickness | | | | |
| Look for oedema | | | | |

## To Finish

| | | | | |
|---|---|---|---|---|
| Review observation chart, including BP. Examine old photographs of patient | | | | |
| Present findings | | | | |

## General

| | | | | |
|---|---|---|---|---|
| Progressed speedily with confidence | | | | |
| Communicates clear instructions to patient | | | | |
| Minimises pain and makes patient feel at ease | | | | |

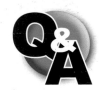

## Questions And Answers for Candidate

### How would you confirm the diagnosis of acromegaly?

- Measure growth hormone levels during an oral glucose tolerance test
- Growth hormone level is not suppressed after consuming the carbohydrate load; there may be a paradoxical rise in growth hormone levels

## Give three causes of tall stature.

- Familial
- Genetic:      Chromosomal e.g. Klinefelter's
                     Overgrowth syndomes e.g. Marfan's Syndrome / Sotos Syndrome
- Endocrine:   Growth hormone-secreting pituitary tumour
                     Precocious puberty
                     Hyperthyroidism
                     Normal variation / Simple obesity

## What complications may arise in a patient with acromegaly? State two.

- Diabetes mellitus or impaired glucose tolerance
- Increased blood pressure and left ventricular hypertrophy
- Cardiomyopathy
- Malignancy, particularly colorectal cancer

The Unofficial Guide to Passing OSCEs: *Candidate Briefings, Patient Briefings and Mark Schemes*

1 // What is the commonest cause of acromegaly?

2 // What drug would be used for the medical therapy of acromegaly?

3 // What is the clinical consequence of excess growth hormone in childhood compared to in adulthood?

4 // Growth hormone causes what to be released from the liver?

5 // What part of the pituitary gland does GnRH act on?

Examination

# Station 21
# THYROID EXAMINATION

*Candidate Briefing:* **Mr. Pryce has recently lost weight, and has profound diarrhoea. He also has developed a lump in his neck. Please examine him and assess his thyroid status.**

## Mark Scheme for Examiner

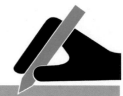

### Introduction

| | | | | |
|---|---|---|---|---|
| Clean hands, introduce self, confirm patient identity and gain consent | | | | |
| Neck adequately exposed | | | | |

### General Inspection

| | | | | |
|---|---|---|---|---|
| Hair, skin, behaviour, build, clothing | | | | |

### Hands

| | | | | |
|---|---|---|---|---|
| Look for thyroid acropatchy, onycholysis, sweatiness, palmar erythema, fine tremor | | | | |
| Feel pulse | | | | |

### Eyes

| | | | | |
|---|---|---|---|---|
| Chemosis, periorbital oedema, erythema, lid retraction | | | | |
| From the side and above assess exophthalmos | | | | |
| Ophthalmoplegia: assess cranial nerves III, IV, VI | | | | |
| Lid lag | | | | |

## Neck Inspection

| | | | | | |
|---|---|---|---|---|---|
| Inspect from front and side | | | | | |
| Scars, hyperaemia, swelling, distended veins | | | | | |
| Inspect whilst the patient sips water | | | | | |
| Inspects whilst the patient sticks tongue out | | | | | |

## Palpation

| | | | | | |
|---|---|---|---|---|---|
| Palpate from behind | | | | | |
| Temperature | | | | | |
| Palpate whilst swallowing | | | | | |
| Palpate whilst sticking out tongue | | | | | |
| Assess any swelling: site, size, shape, consistency, edge, mobility, fluctuance, transillumination, relationship to skin and deep structures | | | | | |
| Lymph nodes: submental, submandibular, anterior chain, supraclavicular, posterior chain, parotid nodes, mastoid nodes, occipital nodes | | | | | |
| Tracheal deviation | | | | | |

## Percussion

| | | | | | |
|---|---|---|---|---|---|
| Sternum | | | | | |

## Auscultation

| | | | | | |
|---|---|---|---|---|---|
| Bruits | | | | | |

## To Finish

| | | | | | |
|---|---|---|---|---|---|
| Review observation chart. Look for pretibial myxoedema, assess tendon reflexes, and assess for proximal myopathy | | | | | |
| Present findings | | | | | |

## General

| Progressed speedily with confidence | | | | | |
|---|---|---|---|---|---|
| Communicates clear instructions to patient | | | | | |
| Minimises pain and makes patient feel at ease | | | | | |

## Questions And Answers for Candidate

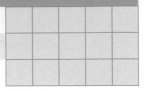

### Name four causes for a thyroid swelling.

| Smooth/diffuse: | Hashimoto's disease |
|---|---|
| | Grave's disease |
| | Iodine deficiency |

| Solitary nodule: | Cyst |
|---|---|
| | Colloid nodule |
| | Adenoma |
| | Carcinoma |
| | Dominant nodule multinodular goitre |

| Multiple nodules: | Multiple cyst |
|---|---|
| | Multinodular goitre |

### Name three signs of hyperthyroidism particularly seen in Graves' disease.

- Eye disease: exophthalmos, ophthalmoplegia
- Pretibial myxoedema
- Thyroid acropachy

## Give three complications of thyrotoxicosis.

- Heart failure
- Angina
- Atrial fibrillation
- Osteoporosis
- Ophthalmopaplegia
- Gynaecomastia
- Thyrotoxic crisis

## Additional Questions to Consider

1 // **In primary hyperthyroidism, what would you expect the thyroid function tests to show?**

2 // **What drug/class of drugs might you prescribe to control symptoms of hyperthyroidism?**

3 // **What other endocrine conditions might be associated with Graves' disease?**

4 // **Is Graves' disease more common in males or females?**

5 // **What initial investigations would you perform in hyperthyroidism?**

# Station 22
# HAEMATOLOGICAL EXAMINATION

*Candidate Briefing:* **Mrs. Hutchison is a 44 year-old lady who reports feeling 'under the weather' over the last few weeks. She has lost considerable weight, bruises more easily than before, and has recently been sweating profusely. Please perform a relevant examination and present your findings.**

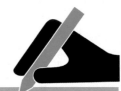

## Mark Scheme for Examiner

### Introduction

| | | | | | |
|---|---|---|---|---|---|
| Clean hands, introduce self, confirm patient identity and gain consent | | | | | |
| Patient adequately exposed | | | | | |

### General Inspection

| | | | | | |
|---|---|---|---|---|---|
| Assess colour (pallor / plethora / jaundice) | | | | | |
| Check for signs of bleeding (purpura / bruising) | | | | | |
| Breathlessness | | | | | |

### Hands

| | | | | | |
|---|---|---|---|---|---|
| Capillary refill time | | | | | |
| Temperature | | | | | |
| Pale skin creases, telangiectasia, kolionychia | | | | | |

The Unofficial Guide to Passing OSCEs: *Candidate Briefings, Patient Briefings and Mark Schemes*

Examination

## Pulse

Rate, rhythm, volume

## Mouth

Lips (angular stomatitis, telangectasia)

Gums (hypertrophy, bleeding)

Tongue (colour, smoothness)

Buccal mucosae (petechiae)

Tonsils

Conjunctivae (pallor, jaundice)

## Fundi

Haemorrhage, engorged veins, papilloedema

## Lymph Nodes of Neck and Axillae

Lymph nodes: submental, submandibular, deep cervical, preauricular, postauricular, occipital, supraclavicular, infraclavicular, axillary

Feel for size, consistency and tenderness in all of the above

## Abdomen

Abdominal examination

Palpate liver and spleen

Inguinal lymph nodes

## Legs

Assess the peripheral circulation (gangrene, arterial supply)

Oedema

## Additional Lymph Nodes

Epitrochlear, axillary, inguinal, femoral

## To Finish

Review observation chart

Present findings

## General

Progressed speedily with confidence

Communicates clear instructions to patient

Minimises pain and makes patient feel at ease

## Questions And Answers for Candidate

### Give two ways to differentiate between an enlarged spleen and a kidney?

- The spleen has a notch, the kidney does not
- The spleen is dull to percussion, the kidney is resonant
- Cannot get between the ribs and spleen, can get fingers over the kidney
- Spleen moves down on inspiration, kidney does not move

## Give three causes of a normocytic anaemia.

- Acute blood loss
- Anaemia of chronic disease
- Bone marrow failure
- Renal failure
- Hypothyroidism
- Haemolysis
- Pregnancy

## What factor is deficient in Haemophillia A?

- Factor VIII

## Additional Questions to Consider

1 // The Hb comes back at 9g / dl. What considerations would you make when deciding whether to give Mr Hutchison a blood transfusion?

2 // In a microcytic anaemia, what additional blood tests might you want to consider?

3 // What are 'blast' cells, and when might they be seen?

4 // How would you investigate a macrocytic anaemia?

5 // What is the difference between a leukaemia and a lymphoma?

# Station 23
# EYE EXAMINATION

*Candidate Briefing:* **Mrs. Baker is an 80 year-old lady and lifelong smoker. She has noticed that her left eyelid has become droopy. Please examine her eyes. You do not need to examine her fundi.**

## Mark Scheme for Examiner

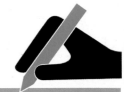

### Introduction

| | | | | | |
|---|---|---|---|---|---|
| Clean hands, introduce self, confirm patient identity and gain consent | | | | | |

### Inspection

| | | | | | |
|---|---|---|---|---|---|
| Glasses, eye asymmetry, ptosis, proptosis, lid lesions, red eyes | | | | | |
| Signs of systemic diseases | | | | | |

### Visual Acuity

| | | | | | |
|---|---|---|---|---|---|
| Each eye in turn, glasses on | | | | | |
| Distance vision (Snellen chart at 6m) | | | | | |
| Check whether this improves with a pinhole | | | | | |
| Test near vision at ~30cm | | | | | |

### Visual fields

| | | | | | |
|---|---|---|---|---|---|
| Test each eye in turn, using a small red object | | | | | |
| Compare patient's field to yours | | | | | |

## Pupillary Reflexes

Direct light reflex

Consensual light reflex

Accommodation reflex

Test for relative afferent papillary defect

## Eye Movements

Examine eye movements noting nystagmus (direction, number of beats) and double vision (including which extraocular muscle might be effected)

## To Finish

Review observation chart. Perform fundoscopy

Present findings

## General

Progressed speedily with confidence

Communicates clear instructions to patient

Minimises pain and makes patient feel at ease

## Name four causes of a red eye.

- Conjunctivitis
- Episcleritis
- Scleritis
- Keratitis or corneal abrasion
- Corneal foreign body
- Dry eyes
- Subconjunctival haemorrhage
- Acute angle-closure glaucoma
- Anterior uveitis

## What might cause an absent red reflex in a baby?

- Congenital cataract
- Retinoblastoma

## What signs might you find to support a diagnosis of Horner's Syndrome?

- Meiosis
- Enophthalmos
- Partial ptosis
- Anhydrosis on affected side

1 // What is nystagmus? When (if ever) is it normal?

2 // If unable to see any letters on a Snellen chart, what else could be used to assess vision?

3 // What pattern of visual loss would be characteristic of age-related macular degeneration?

4 // What is myopia?

5 // Explain how you would test for a relative afferent pupillary defect.

*Candidate Briefing: **Mrs. Mason is an 82 year-old lady who is finding it increasingly difficult to hear. Please examine her ears and present your findings. The tympanic membrane findings are shown in the picture below.***

IMAGE 1: (Chapter 2, Station 24: Unofficial Guide to Passing OSCEs)

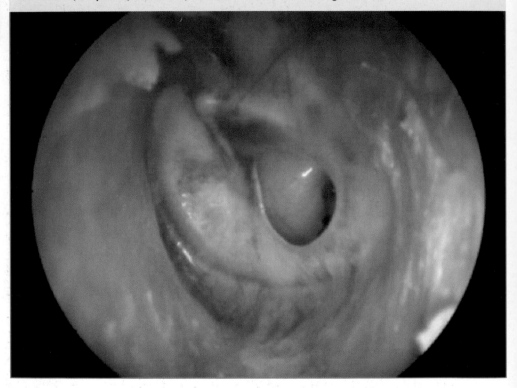

**Additional Images to Practice:**
(follow on the next page)

Examination

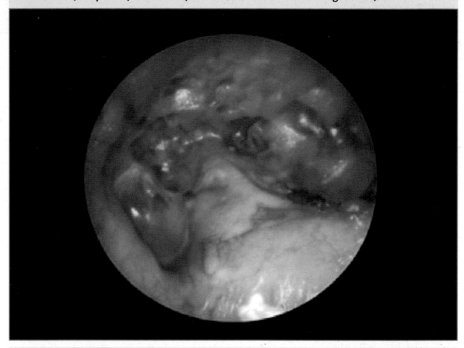

Examination

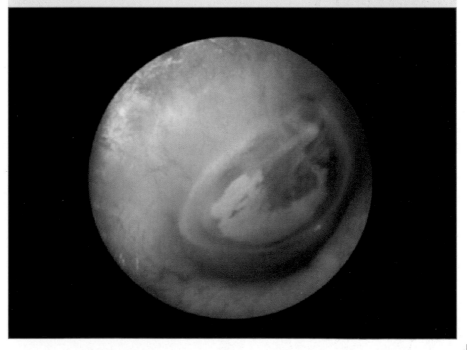

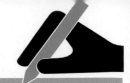

# Mark Scheme for Examiner

## Introduction

| | | | | |
|---|---|---|---|---|
| Clean hands, introduce self, confirm patient identity and gain consent | | | | |

## Examine the External Ear

| | | | | |
|---|---|---|---|---|
| Inspect the pre-auricular area for an endaural incision scar | | | | |
| Inspect the pinna for any lesions | | | | |
| Post-auricular area for a post-auricular incision scar | | | | |
| Palpate the mastoid area for tenderness | | | | |
| Palpate the post-auricular area for evidence of a cochlear implant | | | | |

## Examine the Auditory Meatus and Tympanic Membrane

| | | | | |
|---|---|---|---|---|
| Select appropriate speculum | | | | |
| Check light source and hold appropriately | | | | |
| Get patient to tilt their head, pull the pinna up and back | | | | |
| Ear canal: look for wax and signs of infection | | | | |
| Tympanic membrane: normal/abnormal, location of pathology (pars flaccida/tensa), size of any perforation | | | | |

## Examination of Hearing

| | | | | |
|---|---|---|---|---|
| Whisper test | | | | |
| Rinne's test | | | | |
| Weber's test | | | | |

Examination

## To Finish

| | | | | | |
|---|---|---|---|---|---|
| Review observation chart. Examine the facial nerve. Pure tone audiogram | | | | | |
| Present findings | | | | | |

## General

| | | | | | |
|---|---|---|---|---|---|
| Progressed speedily with confidence | | | | | |
| Communicates clear instructions to patient | | | | | |
| Minimises pain and makes patient feel at ease | | | | | |

---

*Findings on Image 1:*
**'Her left ear has a 10% central perforation in the posterio-inferior quadrant.**

On examination of the external ear, there are no pinna lesions or deformities, no mastoid tenderness, no evidence of previous ear surgery. She wears no hearing aids or implant devices. On examination of the external auditory meatus and tympanic membrane, she has bilaterally dry ears with no mastoid cavities; her right tympanic membrane looks healthy and normal, however her left ear has a 10% central perforation in the posterio-inferior quadrant. This ear was Rinne's negative suggesting conductive hearing loss. There was no lateralisation on Weber's test. Whisper testing was normal in both ears. These findings are consistent with a left tympanic membrane perforation.

Causes for this may be:
1. Perforation secondary to acute otitis media
2. A complication of grommet insertion
3. Barotrauma

**To fully assess the patient's hearing I would like to perform a
pure tone audiogram and a tympanogram.'**

---

### Findings on Image 2:

**Mastoid Cavity:** 'On examination of the external auditory meatus and tympanic membrane, I can see that this is a dry ear with no signs of infection or bleeding. There is an obvious cavity in the superoposterior aspect of the ear canal that is consistent with a mastoid cavity, perhaps indicating previous surgery for a cholesteatoma. The tympanic membrane is intact with a positive light reflex.

*I would like to perform a pure tone audiogram in order to see if there is any conductive hearing loss, which can occur due to ossicular erosion with cholesteatomas'*

### Findings on Image 3:

**Tympanosclerosis:** 'On examination of the external auditory meatus and tympanic membrane, I can see that this is a dry right ear. There is opacification of the tympanic membrane consistent with Tympanosclerosis.

*I would like to perform a tympanogram in order to see if there is reduced motility of the drum, and a pure tone audiogram to see if there is any associated conductive hearing loss.'*

## Questions And Answers for Candidate

## What might cause perforation of the eardrum?

- Otitis media
- Trauma
- Complication of grommet insertion

## Give three complications of otitis media.

- Perforation of the ear drum
- Mastoiditis
- Cholesteatoma
- Labyrinthitis
- Facial paralysis
- Meningitis
- Brain abscess
- Hearing problems
- Developmental problems

## Would Rinne's test be positive or negative in sensorineural deafness?

- Positive i.e. air conduction is greater than bone conduction on the affected side

## Additional Questions to Consider

1 // Would fluid in the middle ear cause a conductive or sensorineural hearing loss?

2 // What is presbycusis, and would it cause a conductive or sensorineural hearing loss?

3 // What is tinnitus? What might cause this?

4 // In Weber's test, in an abnormal ear, would the sound be louder or quieter compared to the normal ear?

5 // What are the typical tympanic membrane changes in otitis media?

Examination

# Station 25
# NEWBORN BABY EXAMINATION

*Candidate Briefing:* **You are the junior doctor covering the postnatal ward. You routinely perform a baby check on baby Barton, who is 12 hours old. He is the first child of a 36 year-old woman, and was delivered by normal vaginal delivery. Combined antenatal screening was not undertaken. Before seeing the baby, the midwife has called your attention to the baby's facial features.**

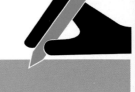

## Mark Scheme for Examiner

### Introduction

| | | | | | |
|---|---|---|---|---|---|
| Clean hands, introduce self, confirm patient identity | | | | | |
| Baby fully undressed | | | | | |

### Head

| | | | | | |
|---|---|---|---|---|---|
| Shape (caput / cephalhaematoma / swelling crossing suture lines) | | | | | |
| Sagittal and coronal suture lines | | | | | |
| Size (measure and plot head circumference) | | | | | |
| Size and shape of anterior and posterior fontanelles | | | | | |
| Check no abnormal facial features (e.g. hypertelorism, micrognathia) | | | | | |
| Eyes – check red reflex | | | | | |
| Mouth: Normal shape, no cleft lip / Exclude tongue-tie / Palpate for cleft palate / Assess suck reflex | | | | | |
| Ears: Ensure normal position / Exclude auricular skin tags and sinuses | | | | | |

## Cardiovascular

Precordium:  Palpate for heaves and thrills
Listen to heart sounds and murmurs
Measure heart rate and rhythm

Palpate femoral pulses

Ensure no cyanosis

## Respiratory

Check no deformities (e.g. pectus excavatum, accessory nipples)

Auscultate

Measure respiratory rate

Check no signs of respiratory distress

## Skin

Examine entire body

Check for birthmarks (e.g. haemangioma, Mongolian blue spots)

Check no rashes

## Abdomen

Palpation (organomegaly, masses)

Herniae (umbilical, inguinal)

Umbilicus – check no infection

Anus – check is patent

Examination

## Genitalia

Check not ambiguous

Males:      Both testes descended
            Penis does not have hypospadias

## Musculoskeletal

Hands/feet:  Polydactyly, syndactyly, palmar creases
             Talipes – positional / fixed?

Spine:       Straight? Sacral dimples? Tufts of hair?

Hips:        Barlow and Ortolani manoeuvres

## Neurological

Reflexes - Moro and grasp

Head lag

Assess tone

Stepping reflex

## To Finish

Review observation chart

Present findings

## General

Progressed speedily with confidence

Communicates clear instructions to patient

Minimises pain and makes patient feel at ease

### Give two cardiac complications associated with Down syndrome?

- Atrioventricular septal defect
- Atrial septal defect
- Ventral septal defect

### What conditions are checked for in the Guthrie test?

- Hypothyroidism
- Sickle cell
- Thalassaemias
- Cystic fibrosis
- MCAD deficiency
- PKU

### What does the APGAR score assess?

- Appearance (blue or pale all over (0 points), pink body with blue extremities (1 point), pink all over (2 points))
- Pulse rate (absent (0 points), <100 (1 point), >100 (2 points))
- Grimace (no response to stimulation (0 points), feeble cry or grimace to stimulation (1 point), cry or pull away to stimulation (2 points))
- Activity (no muscle tone (0 points), some flexion (1 point), good muscle tone (2 points))
- Respiration (absent (0 points), weak and irregular (1 points), strong cry (2 points))

1 // What is the most worrying complication of neonatal jaundice, and how can neonatal jaundice be treated?

2 // What might cause gyaenacomastia in a newborn baby?

3 // What is the normal range of respiratory rate in a neonate?

4 // What would make you concerned about a possible coarctation of the aorta?

5 // What is the average birth weight and head circumference in a newborn baby born at term?

# Chapter 3

# Orthopaedics

# Station 1
# THORACOLUMBAR SPINE

*Candidate Briefing:* **Mr Lasèugue is an 85 year-old gentleman who has recently developed back pain. He is known to have prostate cancer. Please examine his thoracolumbar spine.**

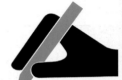

## Mark Scheme for Examiner

### Introduction

| | | | | |
|---|---|---|---|---|
| Clean hands, introduce self, confirm patient identity and gain consent | | | | |
| Adequately exposes patient | | | | |

### Look

| | | | | |
|---|---|---|---|---|
| Gait | | | | |
| With the patient standing, inspects from back and side | | | | |
| Comment on café au lait spots, fat pad / hairy patch, previous scars, muscle spasm, symmetry | | | | |
| Comment on alignment of shoulder / hip / knee / ankle | | | | |
| Comment on thoracic / lumbar curvature | | | | |
| With patient standing with back against wall, comment on whether heels, pelvis, shoulder, occiput simultaneously touch wall | | | | |

## Feel

| T1 to sacrum, and the sacroiliac joints | | | | | |
|---|---|---|---|---|---|
| Paraspinal musculature | | | | | |

## Percuss

| Percuss spine | | | | | |
|---|---|---|---|---|---|

## Move

| Examines flexion of the lumbar spine (including using Schober method) | | | | | |
|---|---|---|---|---|---|
| Examines extension, rotation and lateral flexion (both sides) | | | | | |

## Special Tests

| Straight leg raise (measures angle) | | | | | |
|---|---|---|---|---|---|
| Tibial stretch test | | | | | |
| Femoral stretch test | | | | | |

## General Points

| Presents findings | | | | | |
|---|---|---|---|---|---|
| States would a) perform neurovascular assessment of legs b) perform rectal exam c) examine the joint above and below | | | | | |
| Progressed speedily with confidence | | | | | |
| Communicates clear instructions to patient | | | | | |
| Minimises pain and makes patient feel at ease | | | | | |

Orthopaedics

---

### What are the initial investigations and management of a patient presenting with suspected cauda equina syndrome?

- Analgesia
- White Cell Count and CRP for evidence of infection
- MRI scan of the lumbar spine
- Urgent referral to neurosurgeons and consideration of surgery

---

### Name four red flag symptoms of back pain.

- Onset age >55 or <20 years
- Constant or progressive pain
- Nocturnal pain
- Morning stiffness
- History of carcinoma
- Constitutional symptoms (fevers, unexplained weight loss, night sweats)
- Progressive neurological deficit
- Current or recent infection
- Disturbed gait
- Saddle anaesthesia
- Bladder or bowel dysfunction
- Leg claudication
- Immunosuppression

## Name five causes of lower back pain.

- Degenerative changes
- Trauma
- Tumour
- Infection
- Scoliosis
- Postural pain
- Non spinal pathology
- Spondyloysis / spondylolisthesis
- Psychological component

## Additional Questions to Consider

1 // What is the prevalence of simple back pain?

2 // How is uncomplicated back pain best managed?

3 // What tumours / cancers are associated with spinal pathology?

4 // What infective agents are common in the spine?

5 // What are the different types of scoliosis and how does it present?

# Station 2
# CERVICAL SPINE EXAMINATION

*Candidate Briefing:* **Mr Smith is an 85 year-old gentleman who fell off a ladder. He is complaining of some neck pain. Please examine his cervical spine.**

## Mark Scheme for Examiner

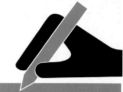

### Introduction

| | | | | |
|---|---|---|---|---|
| Clean hands, introduce self, confirm patient identity and gain consent | | | | |
| Adequately exposes patient | | | | |

### Look

| | | | | |
|---|---|---|---|---|
| Inspects patient from front, side and back | | | | |
| Comments on posture / position of neck / patient | | | | |
| Looks for muscle wasting, scars and lumps | | | | |

### Feel

| | | | | |
|---|---|---|---|---|
| Spinous processes | | | | |
| Facet joints | | | | |
| Paraspinal and trapezius muscles | | | | |
| Crepitus | | | | |
| Around the neck for lymphadenopathy / cervical rib | | | | |

## Move

| | | | | | |
|---|---|---|---|---|---|
| Flexion | | | | | |
| Lateral flexion | | | | | |
| Extension | | | | | |
| Rotation | | | | | |

## Special / Further Tests

| | | | | | |
|---|---|---|---|---|---|
| Lhermitte's Sign | | | | | |
| Examines for thoracic outlet syndrome | | | | | |

## General Points

| | | | | | |
|---|---|---|---|---|---|
| Presents findings | | | | | |
| States would a) perform a neurovascular assessment of the upper limbs and b) full peripheral neurological examination | | | | | |
| Progressed speedily with confidence | | | | | |
| Communicates clear instructions to patient | | | | | |
| Minimises pain and makes patient feel at ease | | | | | |

Orthopaedics

---

## How would you manage a patient with a possible unstable cervical spinal fracture?

- Inline triple immobilisation
- Analgesia
- AP and lateral X-rays of the cervical spine (C1-T1) and peg view
- Discussion with orthopaedics / neurosurgeons
- Further imaging as indicated CT / MRI

---

## What management options are available for C-Spine Injuries?

- Soft Collars: useful for pain relief in minor injuries
- Hard Collars: can be used to treat a variety of injuries
- Gardner-Wells Tongs: provides stability and traction as an acute option
- Halo Ring: an external fixator that provides stability of the c-spine
- Operative fixation

---

## What are the clinical features of cervical spondylosis?

- Neck pain and stiffness
- Gradual onset and worse in the morning
- Radiation of the pain often up the occiput
- May have neurological symptoms such as weakness or altered sensation in one or both arms
- Tender across c-spine and scapulae
- Limited neck movements that are painful

1 // What are the important lines and measurements to look for when assessing a c-spine X-ray?

2 // What fracture patterns are common in the c-spine?

3 // What are the differences between the paediatric and adult c-spine X-ray when assessing for injury?

4 // How do inflammatory arthropathies affect the c-spine?

5 // What congenital abnormalities may occur in the c-spine?

Orthopaedics

# Station 3
# HAND EXAMINATION

*Candidate Briefing:* **Mr Payne is a 50 year-old gentleman who has been suffering from arthritis for the last 10 years. He is finding it progressively more difficult to write and to carry out household tasks with his hands. Please examine his hands and present your findings.**

## Mark Scheme for Examiner

### Introduction

| | | | | |
|---|---|---|---|---|
| Clean hands, introduce self, confirm patient identity and gain consent | | | | |
| Adequately exposes patient | | | | |

### Look

| | | | | |
|---|---|---|---|---|
| Looks at patient as a whole for evidence of systemic disease | | | | |
| Assess both hands together, palms and dorsum | | | | |
| Muscle wasting, skin thinning, swelling, erythema, previous scars, rheumatoid changes, Heberden's nodes, Bouchard's nodes | | | | |
| Nails | | | | |

### Feel

| | | | | |
|---|---|---|---|---|
| Temperature | | | | |
| Muscle wasting | | | | |
| Radial and ulnar pulses | | | | |

| Each joint in turn for tenderness (including wrist and anatomical snuff box) | | | | | |
|---|---|---|---|---|---|
| Palpates for tender nodules and Dupuytren's contractures | | | | | |

## Move

| | | | | | |
|---|---|---|---|---|---|
| Flexion, extension, abduction, adduction of the digits | | | | | |
| Wrist flexion and extension | | | | | |
| Assess radial and ulnar deviation | | | | | |
| Assesses supination and pronation | | | | | |
| Examines both passive and active range of movements | | | | | |
| Assesses hand function e.g pick up an object or undo a button | | | | | |

## Special Tests

| | | | | | |
|---|---|---|---|---|---|
| Phalen's Test | | | | | |
| Tinel's Test | | | | | |
| Assesses tendons individually (FDP, FDS, ED, FPL, EPL, EPB) | | | | | |
| Assesses nerves individually motor and sensory (radial, ulnar, median) | | | | | |

## General Points

| | | | | | |
|---|---|---|---|---|---|
| Presents findings | | | | | |
| States that would a) perform a complete neurological and vascular assessment of the upper limbs b) examine the joints above | | | | | |
| Progressed speedily with confidence | | | | | |
| Examines both sides | | | | | |
| Communicates clear instructions to patient | | | | | |
| Minimises pain and makes patient feel at ease | | | | | |

---

**What are some of the common clinical features in the hand of Rheumatoid Arthritis (5 points)?**

- Symmetrical polyarthritis
- Classically effects MCP joints
- Z thumb deformity
- Boutonniere / Swan-neck deformities
- Raised temperature
- Reduced range of movement
- Palmar erythema
- Wasting of thenar eminence
- Wrist subluxation
- Soft tissue swelling
- Wasting of intrinsic muscles of the hand

---

**What are the specific examinations motor and sensory aspects of the radial, ulnar and median nerves?**

- Median nerve, motor: abduct thumbs
- Median nerve, sensory: palmar aspect of thumb, index, middle and lateral half of ring fingers
- Radial nerve, motor: extension of wrist and fingers
- Radial nerve, sensory: dorsum of 1st webspace
- Ulnar nerve, motor: abduction of the fingers
- Ulnar nerve, sensory: little finger and medial half of ring finger

Orthopaedics

## How does Dupuytren's disease present?

- Progressive contractures of the fingers leading to loss of function
- Thickened cord in the palm of the hand
- Little and ring finger most commonly affected
- Family history
- Similar nodules on the knuckles and feet: Garrod's pads and Ledderhose's Disease

## Additional Questions to Consider

**1 //** How does osteoarthritis affect the hand?

**2 //** Why are scaphoid fractures an important diagnosis not to miss?

**3 //** What is a trigger finger and how does it present?

**4 //** What are the features of a flexor sheath infection?

**5 //** What other infections are common in the hand?

# Station 4
# SHOULDER EXAMINATION

*Candidate Briefing:* **Mr O'Humeral is complaining of pain in and around his right shoulder. Please examine his shoulder.**

## Mark Scheme for Examiner

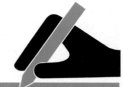

### Introduction

| | | | | |
|---|---|---|---|---|
| Clean hands, introduce self, confirm patient identity and gain consent for history taking | | | | |
| Adequately exposes patient | | | | |

### Look

| | | | | |
|---|---|---|---|---|
| From the front, side and behind | | | | |
| Looks for deformity, swelling, scars, winging of scapula, muscle wasting | | | | |

### Feel

| | | | | |
|---|---|---|---|---|
| From sternoclavicular joint across clavicle to acromioclavicular joint | | | | |
| Palpates acromion, coracoid, scapula spine, and biceps tendon | | | | |

## Move

| | | | | | |
|---|---|---|---|---|---|
| Flexion and extension | | | | | |
| Internal and external rotation | | | | | |
| Abduction and adduction | | | | | |
| Examines both passive and active range of movements | | | | | |
| Assesses function e.g. putting hands behind head | | | | | |

## Special Tests

| | | | | | |
|---|---|---|---|---|---|
| Impingement (painful arc) | | | | | |
| Scarf test | | | | | |
| Bicipital tendinitis | | | | | |
| Shoulder apprehension test | | | | | |
| Examines each of the rotator cuff muscles (supraspinatus, infraspinatus / teres major, subscapularis) | | | | | |
| Winged scapula | | | | | |

## General Points

| | | | | | |
|---|---|---|---|---|---|
| Presents findings | | | | | |
| States would a) perform a neurovascular assessment of the upper limbs b) examine the joints above and below | | | | | |
| Progressed speedily with confidence | | | | | |
| Examines both sides | | | | | |
| Communicates clear instructions to patient | | | | | |
| Minimises pain and makes patient feel at ease | | | | | |

Orthopaedics

### What are the rotator cuff muscles, what is their function and what are their individual actions?

- Supraspinatus, infraspinatus, teres minor, subscapularis
- Provide stability to the glenohumeral joint
- Supraspinatus – first 15 degrees abduction
- Infraspinatus and teres minor – external rotation
- Subscapularis – internal rotation

### What are the management options for a patient with impingement of the shoulder?

- Analgesia including NSAID's
- Physiotherapy and lifestyle modification
- Corticosteroid injections
- Arthroscopy with a subacromial decompression and cuff repair if indicated
- Open repairs may be performed by some surgeons in specific circumstances

## What is a frozen shoulder and how does it present?

- Progressive pain and stiffness in the shoulder
- Presents over several months sometimes following a minor trauma or without a trigger
- Pain can affect sleep and is often severe
- Need to exclude other conditions in the shoulder
- Symptoms usually settle over an 18 month period

## Additional Questions to Consider

1 // What are the types of shoulder dislocation and how are they caused?

2 // What types of shoulder instability are there?

3 // How are fractures of the proximal humerus classified and what is their acute management?

4 // What are the different types of clavicle fractures and how are they managed?

5 // What types of acromioclavicular joint disruption are there?

# Station 5
# HIP EXAMINATION

*Candidate Briefing:* **Mr Trendelenburg has recently fallen. His left lower limb looks shorter than his right, and it is also looks rotated. Please examine his hips.**

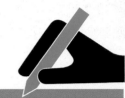

## Mark Scheme for Examiner

### Introduction

| | | | | |
|---|---|---|---|---|
| Clean hands, introduce self, confirm patient identity and gain consent | | | | |
| Adequately exposes patient | | | | |

### Look

| | | | | |
|---|---|---|---|---|
| Compares both sides and looks around bedside for walking aids | | | | |
| Assesses for any deformity, including flexion deformity | | | | |
| Scars, swelling or bruising | | | | |
| Assesses leg length (true and apparent) | | | | |

### Feel

| | | | | |
|---|---|---|---|---|
| Groin crease | | | | |
| Greater trochanter | | | | |
| Warmth | | | | |

## Move

| | | | | | |
|---|---|---|---|---|---|
| Flexion and extension | | | | | |
| External and internal rotation with the hip flexed and extended | | | | | |
| Abduction and adduction | | | | | |
| Active and passive movements | | | | | |

## Special / Further Tests

| | | | | | |
|---|---|---|---|---|---|
| Assesses posture whilst standing (alignment, pelvic tilt), and assesses gait | | | | | |
| Thomas's test | | | | | |
| Trendelenburg test | | | | | |

## General Points

| | | | | |
|---|---|---|---|---|
| Presents findings | | | | |
| States would a) perform a neurovascular assessment of the lower limbs b) examine the joints above and below | | | | |
| Progressed speedily with confidence | | | | |
| Communicates clear instructions to patient | | | | |
| Minimises pain and makes patient feel at ease | | | | |

Orthopaedics

Orthopaedics

### What are the surgical options for the management of a 'neck of femur' fracture?

- Type of operation depends on type of fracture
- Extracapsular fractures can be intertrochanteric or subtrochanteric
- Intertrochanteric – DHS, subtrochanteric – intramedullary nail
- Intracapsular fractures – hemiarthroplasty, total hip replacement or operative fixation

### Which paediatric condition describes hip fracture particularly common to adolescent obese males?

- Slipped upper femoral epiphysis (SUFE)

### How does osteoarthritis of the hip present?

- Progressive pain and loss of function in the hip
- Pain is in the groin, sometimes the buttock or thigh
- Pain at night suggests more severe disease
- Pain on standing from sitting
- May be a history of OA in other joints / family history / previous trauma to the joint

1 // What conditions/treatments can lead to subtrochanteric fractures of the femur specifically?

2 // What is the clinical presentation of a slipped upper femoral epiphysis and how is it best investigated?

3 // What disease processes other than osteoarthritis may cause pain in the 'hip'?

4 // What types of total hip replacement are available for surgeons?

5 // What is the clinical relevance of a Trendelenburg gait?

6 // What are the differences between transient synovitis and septic arthritis of the hip in children?

7 // How would you investigate suspected osteomyelitis?

Orthopaedics

# Station 6
# KNEE EXAMINATION

*Candidate Briefing:* **Mr Smith is a 65 year-old gentleman who is suffering from pain and stiffness in his knees. Examine the knee joints and tell the examiner about any positive clinical findings as you come across them.**

## Mark Scheme for Examiner

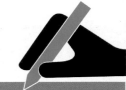

### Introduction

| | | | | | |
|---|---|---|---|---|---|
| Clean hands, introduce self, confirm patient identity and gain consent | | | | | |
| Adequately exposes patient | | | | | |

### Look

| | | | | | |
|---|---|---|---|---|---|
| Looks around the bedside for walking aids, braces or other evidence of disease | | | | | |
| Compares both sides, looking from front side and back, as well as whilst walking | | | | | |
| Looks for deformity (assesses alignment, and comments on any varus / valgus deformity) | | | | | |
| Looks for scars or swelling | | | | | |
| Looks for any muscle wasting (measures thigh circumference) | | | | | |

### Feel

| | | | | | |
|---|---|---|---|---|---|
| For an effusion (either patella tap or sweep test) | | | | | |
| Joint line for tenderness | | | | | |
| Over the patella and the medial and lateral aspects of the knee for point tenderness | | | | | |

| Temperature | | | | | |
|---|---|---|---|---|---|
| Popliteal fossa | | | | | |

## Move

| Assesses both passive and active movements | | | | | |
|---|---|---|---|---|---|
| Feels for crepitus during movements | | | | | |
| Flexion and extension | | | | | |

## Special Tests

| Patellar apprehension test | | | | | |
|---|---|---|---|---|---|
| ACL (Anterior draw test, Lachman test) | | | | | |
| PCL (Posterior draw test / looks for posterior sag) | | | | | |
| Medial and lateral collateral ligaments | | | | | |
| Meniscal injury (McMurray's test) | | | | | |

## End of Examination

| Presents findings | | | | | |
|---|---|---|---|---|---|
| States would a) perform a neurovascular assessment of the lower limbs b) examine the joints above and below | | | | | |
| Progressed speedily with confidence | | | | | |
| Examines both sides | | | | | |
| Communicates clear instructions to patient | | | | | |
| Minimises pain and makes patient feel at ease | | | | | |

Orthopaedics

## How would you investigate and manage osteoarthrtitis of the knee?

- Investigate with weightbearing AP and lateral knee X-rays and possibly arthroscopy
- Non-operative management includes medication and lifestyle changes
- Medications include NSAIDS, simple analgesia, joint injections
- Lifestyle changes include weight loss, stop smoking and physiotherapy
- Surgical options include osteotomies, unicompartmental and total joint replacements

## How does an anterior cruciate ligament injury present and what is the management?

- Trauma to the knee – often a twisting injury
- Immediate swelling often following an audible 'pop' or 'snap'
- Very painful and usually unable to weight bear
- Initial management is non-operative in all except athletes
- Patients who remain symptomatic with instability may require ACL repair which is done open or arthroscopically

## How would you investigate and manage a patient with a dislocated patella?

- Analgesia
- The diagnosis is clinical with a prominent medial femoral condyle
- Reduction is achieved by extending the leg which is usually held in flexion
- Post-reduction X-rays are required to exclude fracture
- Recurrent dislocators may need orthopaedic input and further investigation as to the cause

Orthopaedics

1 // What is the presentation and management of a quadriceps rupture?

2 // What are the different types of meniscal tears and how are they managed?

3 // What are the different types of bursitis of the knee and how are they managed?

4 // What conditions can cause a knee effusion?

5 // What swellings may be found at the back of the knee?

# Station 7
# GALS

*Candidate Briefing: **Mrs Georgeson is a 45 year-old woman who has increasingly stiff joints. Please perform a GALS screen on her and present your findings.***

## Mark Scheme for Examiner

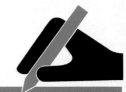

### Introduction

| | | | | |
|---|---|---|---|---|
| Clean hands, introduce self, confirm patient identity and gain consent | | | | |
| Asks all 3 screening questions (pain and stiffness, dressing and walking up and down stairs) | | | | |

### Gait

| | | | | |
|---|---|---|---|---|
| Assess the gait from the front, back and side | | | | |
| Looks at muscle bulk and symmetry, smoothness of movement, turning ability, limp | | | | |
| Comments on any walking aids the patient requires | | | | |

### Arms

| | | | | |
|---|---|---|---|---|
| Looks for muscle wasting or deformity | | | | |
| Asks patient to put arms behind head | | | | |
| Ask patient to stretch out arms, palms facing down, fingers outstretched: inspect dorsum | | | | |
| Ask patient to turn hands over: inspect palm | | | | |
| Ask patient to make a fist | | | | |

| Assess grip strength | | | | | |
| --- | --- | --- | --- | --- | --- |
| Ask patient to bring each finger in turn to meet the thumb of that hand | | | | | |
| Gently squeeze across the MCP joints assessing for tenderness | | | | | |

## Legs

| Looks for muscle wasting or deformity | | | | | |
| --- | --- | --- | --- | --- | --- |
| Tests passive flexion, extension, abduction, adduction of the hip | | | | | |
| Examines the knee for an effusion | | | | | |
| Palpates for any pain around the ankle or forefoot, particularly palpating across the MTP joints | | | | | |

## Spine

| Looks for any scoliosis or kyphosis | | | | | |
| --- | --- | --- | --- | --- | --- |
| Assesses flexion and extension of cervical spine | | | | | |
| Tests for rotation of the thoracic spine | | | | | |
| Assesses temperomandibular joint | | | | | |
| Assesses lumbar flexion | | | | | |
| Asks patient to bend and touch their toes | | | | | |

## End of Examination

| Progressed speedily with confidence | | | | | |
| --- | --- | --- | --- | --- | --- |
| Communicates clear instructions to patient | | | | | |
| Minimises pain and makes patient feel at ease | | | | | |

Orthopaedics

### What are the clinical features of acute gout and how is it best managed?

- Acute onset of pain
- Painful swollen joint most often metatarsophalangeal joint of the big toe
- Joint aspiration will confirm the diagnosis with negative birefringent crystals
- Analgesics including traditionally colchicines although more often NSAIDS
- Steroids in severe cases

### What is hallux valgus and how is it best managed?

- Is a valgus deformity of the big toe often referred to as a 'bunion'
- It is caused by footwear specifically high heeled shoes
- Pain relief and altered footwear
- There are many operations available; all aim to correct the deformity of the great toe

### What are the investigations and management of an achilles tendon rupture?

- Clinical assessment is usually sufficient for the diagnosis
- Ultrasound is useful if diagnosis unclear
- Pain relief, elevation, rest
- All patients should be placed in an equinus (plantar flexion) below knee plaster
- Treatment may be operative or non-operative depending on the patient and the patient's wishes

Orthopaedics

1 // What are the types of pathological gait?

2 // What are the presenting features and management of compressive nerve syndromes of the upper limb?

3 // How does compartment syndrome present and how is it best managed?

4 // What gait is associated with cerebellar disease?

5 // What is tennis elbow and how is it managed?

# Chapter 4

# Communication Skills

# Station 1
# CAPACITY FOR ENDOSCOPY

*Candidate Briefing: You have been asked to see Mr. Cleghorn by the GI team. He has been admitted with haematemesis. He has known alcoholic liver disease. His abbreviated mental test score is currently 6/10. He is refusing to have an endoscopy and says that his symptoms will improve spontaneously. Please explain the endoscopy procedure to him, and assess his capacity to consent for endoscopy.*

*Patient Briefing: Your name is Mr. Cleghorn and you have been admitted to hospital vomiting blood. You have been a heavy drinker in the past and have been told that this has caused liver disease. You have been told by the doctor you need to have an endoscopy however you have been refusing this procedure as you do not think it is necessary and believe that your symptoms will improve spontaneously.*

A doctor is going to come to speak to you about the endoscopy and explain the risks, benefits and alternatives. You have been drinking alcohol heavily today, are currently confused and not orientated in time or place. Because of your confusion you are unable to retain most of the information the doctor tells you. You remain adamant that you do not want an endoscopy but when you are pressed by the doctor you cannot explain the reason for doing the endoscopy and the associated risks and benefits.

*You repeatedly say you do not want the procedure but cannot give a coherent answer as to why this is the case.*

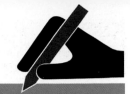

# Mark Scheme for Examiner

## Introduction

| | | | | |
|---|---|---|---|---|
| Clean hands, introduce self, confirm patient identity | | | | |
| Check identity of others in the room and confirm that the patient is happy for them to be present | | | | |
| Establish current patient knowledge and concerns | | | | |

## Explaining an Endoscopy

| | | | | |
|---|---|---|---|---|
| Explain the procedure (describe endoscope, explain use of sedation) and what information will be gained from a endoscopy | | | | |
| Explain the need to sometimes take photographs, tissue samples and give treatment as necessary | | | | |

## Complications of an Endoscopy

| | | | | |
|---|---|---|---|---|
| Sore throat, after effects of sedation, perforation, aspiration, bleeding, reaction to sedation | | | | |

## Contextualise the Information and Explain Alternatives

| | | | | |
|---|---|---|---|---|
| Explain reason for performing the endoscopy (including diagnosis and potential to give treatment) | | | | |
| Advise that you are recommending this procedure | | | | |
| Explore the patient's concerns and anxieties | | | | |
| Explain the alternatives and what the consequences of not having this procedure might be | | | | |

Comm Skills

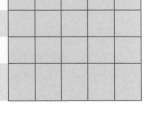

## Assessing Capacity

| | | | | | |
|---|---|---|---|---|---|
| Check that the patient understands the information | | | | | |
| Assess evidence of reason and deliberation, acting on a set of consistent and clear values | | | | | |
| Give the patient the opportunity to communicate back their decision | | | | | |

## Finishing the Consultation

| | | | | | |
|---|---|---|---|---|---|
| Elicit patient concerns or questions | | | | | |
| Summarise back to the patient | | | | | |
| Thank patient and close consultation | | | | | |

## General Points

| | | | | | |
|---|---|---|---|---|---|
| Check patient understands regularly, and offer information leaflets | | | | | |
| Maintain good eye contact and engage with patient | | | | | |
| Avoid medical jargon | | | | | |
| Polite to patient | | | | | |

## Questions And Answers for Candidate

**Do you think this patient has capacity to make the decision regarding having an endoscopy?**

- Based on the patient briefing given, the patient is unable to retain the information given to him long enough to weigh up the risks and benefits of an endoscopy, as well as the alternatives. The patient therefore does not have capacity to make this decision.

## Can you list some of the principles of the Mental Capacity Act (2005) designed to protect and also assist the individual?

- A person must be assumed to have capacity unless it is established that they lack it
- A person is not to be treated as unable to make a decision unless all practical steps have been taken to help them to do so, and without success
- A person must not be treated as unable to make a decision merely because they make an unwise decision
- Any act done or decision made using the Act on behalf of an individual who lacks capacity must be made in their best interests
- Before resorting to the Act, you should see if the purpose for which it is needed can be achieved in some other manner that is less restrictive on the individual's rights or freedom

## What is delirium tremens?

- An acute episode of delirium caused by alcohol withdrawal or abstinence (following habitual excessive drinking), involving tremors, hallucinations, anxiety, and disorientation

## Additional Questions to Consider

1 // What is a delusion?

2 // What is a hallucination?

3 // What are the questions asked in the CAGE screening questionnaire and what do these screen for?

4 // What prognostic scoring tools do you know of for GI bleeds?

5 // Can you tell me some of the differences between the Mental Health Act and the Mental Capacity Act, or when you might use one rather than the other?

*Candidate Briefing: **Mrs. Frederick has attended a GP clinic and is asking for an HIV test. Establish whether she is at low or high risk for HIV. Please explore the risks and benefits of HIV testing.***

*Patient Briefing: **Your name is Mrs. Frederick and you have attended a GP clinic asking for an HIV test. You had an episode of unprotected intercourse recently and want to make sure you have not contracted HIV.***

You are married to your husband and you are heterosexual. Your last sexual contact was one week ago with a man from work who is known to be sexually promiscuous. You had vaginal intercourse only but did not use a condom. You are not aware of this man having HIV.

Otherwise your previous sexual contact was with your husband 2 weeks ago. You had vaginal intercourse only and did not use a condom. You have been married to your husband for 3 years and have regular vaginal sexual intercourse without a condom. You are not aware of your husband having HIV. You have not had any other sexual contacts. You have never had sex with a prostitute, sex abroad or been sexually assaulted. You have never had an invasive procedure in non-sterile conditions, a blood transfusion or abused drugs intravenously. You do not have any sexually transmitted infections (last checked 6 months ago) and have not had any problems with other infections.

You believe that an HIV test is performed as a blood test. You know that AIDS is linked to HIV. You do not want further in-depth counseling regarding the implications of the result at present. You do not feel that you can discuss your most recent sexual encounter with your husband or any of your friends.

***Your main concern is that you might have caught HIV and wish to get the test over with as soon as possible.***

Comm Skills

## Mark Scheme for Examiner

## Introduction

| | | | | |
|---|---|---|---|---|
| Clean hands, introduce self, confirm patient identity | | | | |
| Check identity of others in the room and confirm that the patient is happy for them to be present | | | | |
| Warn patient some questions may be embarrassing | | | | |
| Inform patient that all answers will be kept confidential | | | | |

## Establish Current Patient Knowledge and Concerns

| | | | | |
|---|---|---|---|---|
| Clarify why the patient has attended the clinic and requested an HIV test, elicit patient concerns | | | | |
| Ask whether the patient minds discussing the issues surrounding HIV testing | | | | |

## Assess HIV Risk

| | | | | |
|---|---|---|---|---|
| Sexual orientation – if the patient is male must assess if any episodes of same-sex relationships have occurred | | | | |
| Type of sexual contact – must establish if anal intercourse has occurred since last HIV testing (if appropriate) | | | | |
| Number of partners (and number known to be HIV positive or at high risk), condom usage | | | | |
| Sex with a prostitute (paid for sex), sex abroad (including country of origin, gender of partner, type of sex) | | | | |
| Sexual assault | | | | |
| Invasive procedures in non-sterile conditions | | | | |
| Other sexually transmitted infections | | | | |
| Blood transfusion (including where and when), intravenous drug abuse | | | | |
| Any other health problems (opportunistic infections, immunocompromised states) | | | | |

Comm Skills

## Explaining an HIV Test

| | | | | | |
|---|---|---|---|---|---|
| Clarify patient's understanding of an HIV test | | | | | |
| Explain testing for antibodies against the HIV (virus) using a blood sample | | | | | |
| Explain AIDS as being a result of HIV | | | | | |
| Explain 4th generation testing at six weeks | | | | | |
| Explain the need for repeat testing at 3 months | | | | | |
| Offer in-depth counseling to discuss the implications of the test result | | | | | |
| Enquire about a support network | | | | | |

## Finishing the Consultation

| | | | | | |
|---|---|---|---|---|---|
| Elicit patient concerns or questions | | | | | |
| Summarise back to the patient | | | | | |
| Arrange a follow up appointment or offer your contact details | | | | | |
| Thank patient and close consultation | | | | | |

## General Points

| | | | | | |
|---|---|---|---|---|---|
| Check patient understands regularly, and offer information leaflets | | | | | |
| Maintain good eye contact and engage with patient | | | | | |
| Avoid medical jargon | | | | | |
| Polite to patient | | | | | |

Comm Skills

---

### What do you understand by the sensitivity and the specificity of a test?

- The sensitivity of a HIV test is the percentage of results that will be positive when HIV is present (i.e. sensitive enough to pick it up)
- The specificity of a HIV test is the percentage of results that will be negative when HIV is not present (i.e. specific for HIV and nothing else)

---

### How do modern tests detect HIV?

- They detect antibodies, antigens or nucleic acid (RNA)
- Most laboratories use at least two of these, blood banks tend to use all three

---

### What advice would you give a mother with HIV with regard to feeding her new born baby?

- Breast feeding should be avoided (though this is a more difficult decision if, particularly in the developing world, access to clean water might be an issue)

Comm Skills

1 // What is post-exposure prophylaxis?

2 // What other sexually transmitted infections might you screen for?

3 // What do you understand by the term "informed consent"?

4 // With reference to HIV exposure and testing, what is the "window period"?

5 // Name a method of monitoring HIV progression, or indeed, response to treatment, in a patient with HIV.

# Station 3
# AUTOPSY CONSENT

*Candidate Briefing: Mrs. Parker died last week. You are talking to her daughter. The cause of death was pneumonia. A number of abdominal lesions were noted on CT scanning, which are not thought to be related to the cause of death, but are of unknown origin. The family and medical team are interested to explore this further and your consultant has asked you to get authorisation for a hospital autopsy.*

*Relative Briefing: Your name is Miss Parker and your mother Mrs. Parker died last week. You were aware that she had pneumonia but the doctors had also told you that they had found some lesions in her tummy on a scan.*

You are not aware of your mother ever expressing any views on having an autopsy, and you and the rest of the family wish to know if these lesions were cancer and if so, if there was any increased risk to yourself or other family members of also getting this cancer. You do not know what an autopsy involves but are concerned that your mother's organs may be taken for research purposes. You also wish to have an open casket funeral and want to know if an autopsy will lead to disfiguration of the body.

*If the doctor is able to answer all of your questions and reassure you, you will be happy to consent for the autopsy.*

## Introduction

| | | | | | |
|---|---|---|---|---|---|
| Cleans hands, find suitable location, introduces self, confirms relative's identity | | | | | |
| Check identity of others in the room and confirm that the relative is happy for them to be present, establish if they would like anyone else present | | | | | |
| Establish relative's current knowledge and concerns | | | | | |

## The Autopsy

| | | | | | |
|---|---|---|---|---|---|
| Explain why you are seeking authorisation for an autopsy and what questions you are hoping to answer | | | | | |
| Establish whether the patient had ever expressed views on having an autopsy | | | | | |
| Explain what the autopsy involves | | | | | |
| Explain the possibility of a full or limited autopsy | | | | | |
| Explain the occasional need to retain tissue or organs | | | | | |
| Explain that organs will not be retained without permission | | | | | |
| Explain that an open casket funeral will still be possible if desired by the family | | | | | |
| Explain that permission for the autopsy can be refused | | | | | |
| Explain that permission can be withdrawn at any time up to the autopsy itself | | | | | |

## Finishing the Consultation

| | | | | | |
|---|---|---|---|---|---|
| Elicit relative concerns or questions | | | | | |
| Arrange a follow up appointment (as necessary) or offer your contact details | | | | | |
| Thank relative and close consultation | | | | | |

## General Points

| | | | | | |
|---|---|---|---|---|---|
| Check the relative understands regularly, and offer information leaflets | | | | | |
| Maintain good eye contact and engage with the relative | | | | | |
| Avoid medical jargon | | | | | |
| Polite and empathetic to relative | | | | | |

## Questions And Answers for Candidate

### What details must be recorded when gaining consent for a post mortem (name four)?

- Whether the autopsy will be full or limited
- Whether organs may be retained for detailed examination
- Whether tissue samples may be used for teaching, quality assurance, public health surveillance or clinical audit
- Whether tissue samples may be used for research
- Choice of disposal of retained organs
- Name, signature and details of relative
- Name, signature and details of person taking consent

### Under what circumstances would consent for autopsy not be required?

- The coroner (or Procurator Fiscal) is required by law to establish the cause of death where a death is suspicious, sudden or of an unknown cause
- If they request an autopsy, then consent will neither be sought nor required

## Who can request a post mortem examination or autopsy?

- A doctor, a coroner (or Procurator Fiscal), or sometimes a partner or relative of the patient may all request a post mortem examination
- The examination may be limited to specific areas of the body

## Additional Questions to Consider

**1 //** What is an inquest?

**2 //** List some of the circumstances when you might refer a death to the coroner.

**3 //** What is the estimate of errors on death certification later revealed by post mortem examination?

**4 //** What is a limited autopsy, and why might this be performed?

**5 //** What are the commonest causes of death in the UK?

Comm Skills

# Station 4
# HERNIA REPAIR

*Candidate Briefing:* **Mr. Penneck has recently been diagnosed with an inguinal hernia. Please explain to him what management options are available for him. Please explain to him the risks and benefits of surgical repair of the hernia.**

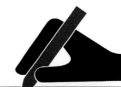

*Patient Briefing:* **Your name is Mr. Penneck and you have recently been diagnosed with an inguinal hernia. You have come to see the doctor today to discuss treatment options.**

You have been experiencing a dragging pain in your groin and noticed a swelling over the last month. You have been told by your GP that you have an inguinal hernia but you are not sure what this actually means. You do not know much about what the treatment options are, but you are keen to see if surgery is possible to remove the hernia and improve your pain.

*You have never had surgery before. However you are anxious because an uncle died after having a blood clot in the lungs post emergency surgery for a perforated duodenal ulcer.*

## Mark Scheme for Examiner

### Introduction

| | | | | |
|---|---|---|---|---|
| Cleans hands, introduces self, confirms patient identity | | | | |
| Check identity of others in the room and confirm that the patient is happy for them to be present | | | | |
| Establish current patient knowledge and concerns | | | | |

## Preparation

| | | | | | |
|---|---|---|---|---|---|
| Explain reason for consultation | | | | | |
| Explain what a hernia is (using diagrams if necessary) | | | | | |
| Explain complications of a hernia (pain, strangulation, bowel obstruction) | | | | | |

## Treatment Options

| | | | | | |
|---|---|---|---|---|---|
| Explain treatment options (conservative vs. surgery) | | | | | |
| Explain surgery can be open or laparoscopic | | | | | |
| Explain what an open repair involves | | | | | |
| Explain what a laparoscopic repair involves (including potential need to convert to open repair) | | | | | |

## Risks of Surgery

| | | | | | |
|---|---|---|---|---|---|
| Infection | | | | | |
| Bleeding | | | | | |
| Post-operative urinary retention (and need for a catheter) | | | | | |
| Area of skin numbness | | | | | |
| Testicular pain | | | | | |
| Chronic abdominal or scrotal pain | | | | | |
| Recurrence of the hernia | | | | | |

## Alternatives to Surgery

| | | | | | |
|---|---|---|---|---|---|
| Explain conservative management and reasons why you would operate on a hernia | | | | | |
| Explain the option of wearing a sling / truss / belt | | | | | |
| Explain the need to treat risk factors for the development of herniae | | | | | |

## Finishing the Consultation

| | | | | |
|---|---|---|---|---|
| Elicit patient concerns or questions | | | | |
| Summarise back to the patient | | | | |
| Arrange a follow up appointment (as necessary) or offer your contact details | | | | |
| Thank patient and close consultation | | | | |

## General Points

| | | | | |
|---|---|---|---|---|
| Check patient understands regularly, and offer information leaflets | | | | |
| Maintain good eye contact and engage with patient | | | | |
| Avoid medical jargon | | | | |
| Polite to patient | | | | |

## Questions And Answers for Candidate

### What are the borders of the inguinal canal?

- The inguinal canal runs from the deep inguinal ring to the superficial inguinal ring and is cylindrical with a roof, a floor, an anterior wall and a posterior wall
- Roof – transversus abdominus, internal oblique and medial crus of external oblique
- Floor – inguinal ligament, lacunar ligament and iliopubic tract
- Anterior wall – aponeurosis of external oblique, internal oblique (lateral 1/3 of canal) and superficial inguinal ring (medial 1/3 of canal)
- Posterior wall – transversalis fascia, conjoint tendon (medial 1/3 of canal), deep ring (lateral 1/3 of canal)

## What types of inguinal hernia repair exist?

- Open repair and laparoscopic repair

## Additional Questions to Consider

1 // Are femoral hernias commoner in men or women?

2 // Which type of hernia is commoner in women, inguinal or femoral?

3 // What signs might you expect on examination if the hernia has led to an obstruction and perforation?

4 // What are the advantages of laparoscopic surgery over open repair?

5 // What is a mesh and why are they used?

# Station 5
# BLOOD TRANSFUSION REACTION

*Candidate Briefing: You are on the phone to a ward nurse who has called you urgently about a patient. The patient started a blood transfusion 2 hours ago. The patient's temperature is now 37.7°C, blood pressure is 99/60 and the patient is anxious. Explore this further on the phone and identify what you would like the nurse to do, and what you are going to do to further manage this patient.*

*Notes on this case: This case is a good example where it is important to give clear instructions to the nurse on the telephone before going to assess the patient and decide if they are having a transfusion reaction.*

In view of the fact that the transfusion started 2 hours ago, ABO incompatibility is less likely as the patient would have become unwell far sooner. A rise in temperature 2 hours into a blood transfusion would lead you to consider a non-haemolytic febrile transfusion reaction. This can be treated either by slowing the transfusion or by stopping the transfusion depending on the degree of concern. Paracetamol would be administered regardless. Whenever you are unsure, the safest practice is to stop the transfusion.

*Nurse's briefing: You are the nurse on ward 11 and you think that one of your patients is having a transfusion reaction. The patient is called Mr. Jones and his transfusion was started 2 hours ago. He was initially well but now his temperature is 37.7°C, blood pressure is 99/60 and the patient is anxious.*

You have called the doctor for advice and want to know if he will come to review the patient. When asked you confirm the patient details as Mr. Jones, hospital number: D293430, date of birth: 2/3/1945. Mr. Jones has a diagnosis of myelodysplastic syndrome and attends for blood transfusions every month. His past medical history includes angina and heart failure. His last haemoglobin was 76g/L and he has come in for a 3 unit blood transfusion. He started his first unit of blood 2 hours ago but has become anxious and his observations have changed. You do not feel the patient is peri-arrest at present.

The current observations are temperature: 37.7°C, blood pressure: 99/60, heart rate: 105bpm, respiratory rate: 22 breaths/minute and oxygen saturations: 93% on air. The observations before the transfusion started were as follows: temperature: 36.6°C, blood pressure 105/66, heart rate: 75bpm, respiratory rate: 16, oxygen saturations: 99% on air.

The patient was feeling anxious so you repeated his observations. When you saw that they had significantly changed, you decided to call the doctor straight away to see if the transfusion needed to be stopped. You have not implemented any management as yet without the instruction of the doctor and have not asked the patient if they have any other symptoms.

Comm Skills

**Your main questions to the doctor are**
- Should the transfusion be stopped?
- What else does the doctor want you to do?
- Will the doctor come to review the patient to see if he needs any medication?
- How long will the doctor be before he reviews the patient?

*You are trained in taking bloods. You would like to be reassured that the doctor considers this a high priority review.*

## Mark Scheme for Examiner

### Introduction

| | | | | | |
|---|---|---|---|---|---|
| Introduce yourself giving your name and job title | | | | | |
| Confirm where the nurse is calling from | | | | | |
| Confirm the patient's identity | | | | | |
| Clarify the current situation and the nurses concerns | | | | | |

### Ascertain How Urgently You Need to See the Patient

| | | | | | |
|---|---|---|---|---|---|
| If the patient is peri-arrest advise the nurse to call the crash team | | | | | |
| Ask for the patient's current observations (temperature, blood pressure, pulse, respiratory rate, oxygen saturations, urine output) | | | | | |
| Ascertain whether there has been a change in any of the patient's observations compared to before transfusion | | | | | |
| Ask if the patient currently has any symptoms | | | | | |
| Clarify the background and the reason for transfusion | | | | | |
| Ask whether the blood is still running | | | | | |
| Find out what management the nursing staff have implemented (e.g. started IV fluids) | | | | | |

## Management in the Case of a Reaction
(directed to nurse)

| | | | | | |
|---|---|---|---|---|---|
| Stop the transfusion | | | | | |
| Start intravenous fluids using a clean giving set through the same cannula (to keep it open) | | | | | |
| Give oxygen if saturations < 94% | | | | | |
| Check the blood pack and patient details | | | | | |
| Administer 1g paracetamol stat | | | | | |
| Take blood (if trained) for FBC, U&Es, Group and Save, Coagulation screen | | | | | |
| Phone the blood bank to inform them of situation | | | | | |
| Consider preparing a trolley for urethral catheter insertion (in case this is required after you have reviewed the patient) | | | | | |

## Finishing the Consultation

| | | | | | |
|---|---|---|---|---|---|
| Summarise what you have discussed | | | | | |
| Inform the nurse you will come to review the patient as a priority and tell them how long you will be; ask them to rebleep you if anything gets worse | | | | | |

## General Points

| | | | | | |
|---|---|---|---|---|---|
| Elicit patient and nurse concerns or questions | | | | | |
| Calm and reassuring manner | | | | | |

Comm Skills

## How would you treat an anaphylactic reaction to blood?

- Stop transfusion
- Adrenaline 0.5mg (0.5ml of 1:1000) IM if hypotensive or if there is presence of angioedema
- Intravenous fluid challenge (e.g. 500ml over 15 minutes) if hypotensive
- Hydrocortisone 200mg IV
- Chlorphenamine 10mg IV
- Salbutamol nebuliser 5mg stat if bronchospasm present

## What are the blood groups, and which is the most common worldwide?

- The groups are A, B, AB and O
- The most common worldwide is blood group O

## How would you confirm, at the bedside, that you are about to connect the correct blood component to correct patient?

The UK BTS guidelines recommend that:
- I ask the patient to state their first name, surname and date of birth
- I check that the ID details match the patient's wrist band
- I check that the ID details match the compatibility label on the blood product
- I check that the blood group and donation number on the product label and compatibility label are identical
- I repeat all these checks for each product transfused

1 // What is the Rhesus factor? Why is this important to know about during pregnancy?

2 // How are blood groups inherited?

3 // What is the universal donor?

4 // What group is the universal recipient?

5 // What is the average circulating volume of blood in an adult?

# Station 6
# WARFARIN COUNSELLING

*Candidate Briefing: Mr. Jacobs is a 70-year-old gentleman recently diagnosed with atrial fibrillation. He had been sent to your cardiology clinic, with a view to potentially starting warfarin therapy. Counsel him about warfarin therapy and its implications.*

*Patient Briefing: You are 70 years old and your name is Mr. Jacobs. You have recently been diagnosed with atrial fibrillation and you have been sent to the cardiology clinic with a view to potentially starting warfarin therapy.*

You have heard of warfarin therapy as one of your neighbours used to take warfarin. You report that they often had to go for blood tests and had restrictions on their diet. You enjoy alcohol, and drink regularly. You have been told that you have an irregular heart beat but you do not know why the doctor wants you started on warfarin. You are concerned that starting warfarin is going to have a big impact on your life and you are wondering whether it is going to be worth all of the trouble.

*If the doctor is able to explain the indications for warfarin clearly and the impact it will have on your life you will agree to start warfarin therapy.*

## Mark Scheme for Examiner

### Introduction

| | | | | | |
|---|---|---|---|---|---|
| Cleans hands, introduces self, confirms patient identity | | | | | |
| Check identity of others in the room and confirm that the patient is happy for them to be present | | | | | |
| Establish current patient knowledge and concerns | | | | | |

The Unofficial Guide to Passing OSCEs: *Candidate Briefings, Patient Briefings and Mark Schemes*

## Approach to Counseling

| | | | | | |
|---|---|---|---|---|---|
| Explain to patient that you want to start warfarin | | | | | |
| Ask if the patient has heard of warfarin before | | | | | |
| Explain warfarin's effect (to thin the blood) | | | | | |
| Explain why you are recommending that the patient takes warfarin, referring to the risk of stroke | | | | | |

## Impact of Warfarin on the Patient's Life

| | | | | | |
|---|---|---|---|---|---|
| Explain the interaction of warfarin with certain foods | | | | | |
| Explain the interaction of warfarin with alcohol | | | | | |
| Explain the interaction of warfarin with other medications | | | | | |
| Explain the need to avoid contact sports | | | | | |

## Warfarin Dosing

| | | | | | |
|---|---|---|---|---|---|
| Explain that all patient's require a different dose of warfarin and that the dose can vary | | | | | |
| Explain monitoring of the INR | | | | | |
| Explain that warfarin should be taken at the same time each day (ideally 6pm) | | | | | |
| Explain the different strengths of warfarin tablets | | | | | |
| Explain the anticoagulation book the patient will be given | | | | | |

## Warnings

| | | | | | |
|---|---|---|---|---|---|
| Inform patient to watch out for bleeding or bruising | | | | | |
| Action to take in the event of bleeding or bruising | | | | | |

Comm Skills

## Finishing the Consultation

| | | | | | |
|---|---|---|---|---|---|
| Elicit patient concerns or questions | | | | | |
| Summarise back to the patient | | | | | |
| Arrange a follow up appointment (as necessary) or offer your contact details | | | | | |
| Thank patient and close consultation | | | | | |

## General Points

| | | | | | |
|---|---|---|---|---|---|
| Check patient understands regularly, and offer information leaflets | | | | | |
| Maintain good eye contact and engage with patient | | | | | |
| Avoid medical jargon | | | | | |
| Polite to patient | | | | | |

## Questions And Answers for Candidate

### Give four examples of drugs that can decrease the INR?

- Vitamin K
- Chronic alcohol intake
- Azathioprine
- Rifampicin
- Oral contraceptive pill
- St John's Wort
- Hormone replacement therapy

## What exactly is the INR?

- INR stands for International Normalised Ratio
- It is a measure of the patient's prothrombin time (PT) compared to a normal (or control) PT taking into account the type of analytical system employed so as to standardise results

## What are the names of the pathways in the coagulation cascade and which does warfarin affect?

- The intrinsic pathway, the extrinsic pathway and the final common pathway
- Warfarin affects the extrinsic pathway

## Additional Questions to Consider

1 // Can you name some alternatives to warfarin therapy?

2 // What clotting factors does warfarin affect?

3 // List some ways of reversing warfarin?

4 // Please name some other indications for warfarin therapy.

5 // What complications of warfarin should you advise the patient to watch out for?

# Station 7
## OPIATE COUNSELING

*Candidate Briefing: **Mr. Smith is suffering from severe pain. He has a diagnosis of inoperable pancreatic cancer. You have found it difficult to control his pain, and now feel his analgesia should be increased. Please counsel him on the risks and benefits of morphine therapy, and discuss other adjuncts to improve his symptoms.***

*Patient Briefing: **Your name is Mr. Smith and you have been suffering from severe pain. You were diagnosed with inoperable pancreatic cancer recently and the doctors have been finding it difficult to control your pain.***

The nurse has informed you that one of the doctors is coming to speak to you about starting morphine. You are apprehensive about this as you are concerned that you will become addicted to morphine. You are also worried about all of the possible side effects and whether these will make things even worse. You are wondering whether there is anything else that might help you.

*If the doctor is able to answer all of your questions and reassure you regarding addiction you will be happy to start morphine therapy.*

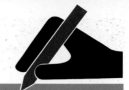

## Mark Scheme for Examiner

## Introduction

Cleans hands, introduces self, confirms patient identity

Check identity of others in the room and confirm that the patient is happy for them to be present. Establish if patient would like anyone else present

Establish current patient knowledge and concerns

## Patient Concerns

Explain to the patient that you would recommend starting morphine for pain control

Establish patient concerns regarding morphine therapy

Address concerns regarding addiction

Reassure that morphine will not hasten death

Reassure that taking morphine now will not mean that it won't work later

## Morphine Therapy

Discuss formulations of morphine (short and long acting)

Discuss different routes of administration

## Side Effects of Morphine

Constipation: discuss the use of laxatives

Nausea: discuss the use of anti-emetics

Drowsiness: sometimes a dose reduction will be required or a different formulation

Myoclonus: sometimes a dose reduction will be required or other medications can be given to counteract this (e.g. midazolam)

Comm Skills

| Hallucinations | | | | | |
|---|---|---|---|---|---|
| Tolerance | | | | | |

## Other Approaches (discusses at least three)

| Palliative care team involvement | | | | | |
|---|---|---|---|---|---|
| TENS machine | | | | | |
| Acupuncture | | | | | |
| Aromatherapy | | | | | |
| Relaxation techniques | | | | | |
| Emotional and spiritual support | | | | | |

## Finishing the Consultation

| Elicit patient concerns or questions | | | | | |
|---|---|---|---|---|---|
| Summarise back to the patient | | | | | |
| Arrange a follow up appointment (as necessary) or offer your contact details | | | | | |
| Thank patient and close consultation | | | | | |

## General Points

| Check patient understands regularly, and offer leaflets | | | | | |
|---|---|---|---|---|---|
| Maintain good eye contact and engage with patient | | | | | |
| Avoid medical jargon | | | | | |
| Polite to patient | | | | | |

### What are the symptoms and signs of opiate toxicity (up to three marks)?

- Reduced consciousness
- Respiratory depression
- Pinpoint pupils

### What is the difference between an opiate and an opioid?

- The term opiate is limited to natural alkaloids derived directly from the opium poppy
- Opioids are psychoactive chemicals that bind to the opioid receptors in the nervous system (and elsewhere). They include all opiates and also synthetically derived chemicals

### What is meant by the term tolerance?

- Tolerance is a neuro-adaptive process resulting in reduced drug effects through receptor desensitisation

## Additional Questions to Consider

1 // Define the terms agonist, partial-agonist and competitive inhibition.

2 // What is an endorphin?

# Station 8: Lifestyle Advice: POST MYOCARDIAL INFARCTION

*Candidate Briefing: Mr. Smith is about to be discharged home from hospital. He was admitted after having a heart attack. Please explore why he was at risk for developing heart disease. Explore what lifestyle measures could be adopted to reduce his risk of another event.*

*Patient Briefing: Your name is Mr. Smith and you have recently suffered a heart attack. You are pleased to hear that you have recovered well and should be discharged home soon. The nurse informs you that the doctor would like to come to talk to you about your lifestyle to prevent further problems with your heart.*

When asked by the doctor you admit that prior to coming into hospital you did not lead the healthiest lifestyle. This heart attack has been a real shock and you are keen to change your ways to prevent this happening again. You admit that you have smoked about 20 cigarettes a day for the last 40 years. Whilst in hospital you have been told that you have both high cholesterol and high blood pressure. You admit that you could lose some weight – you currently weigh about 100kg and your height is 1.7m. The nurse told you that this makes your BMI about 35. You drink on average 3 pints of lager every evening and admit that you need to cut down. You do not know how much salt is in your diet but report that you often eat takeaways or have fried food.

*The biggest limitation for you is that you do not know how to cook, and there is no one there to help. You do not do any regular exercise but report that you do not have any extra stress in your life, apart from the recent heart attack!*

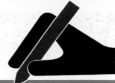

## Mark Scheme for Examiner

## Introduction

| | | | | | |
|---|---|---|---|---|---|
| Clean hands, introduce self, confirm patient identity | | | | | |
| Check identity of others in the room and confirm that the patient is happy for them to be present, establish if patient would like anyone else present | | | | | |
| Establish current patient knowledge and concerns | | | | | |
| Explain to the patient that you have come to talk to them about lifestyle advice after their heart attack | | | | | |

## Establish the Patient's Risks Factors for Heart Disease

| | | | | | |
|---|---|---|---|---|---|
| Smoking | | | | | |
| Dyslipidaemia | | | | | |
| Hypertension | | | | | |
| Diabetes | | | | | |
| Obesity | | | | | |
| Excess alcohol intake | | | | | |
| Excess salt intake | | | | | |
| Lack of exercise | | | | | |
| Environmental stress | | | | | |

Comm Skills

## Lifestyle Advice

| | | | | | |
|---|---|---|---|---|---|
| Weight loss | | | | | |
| Alcohol reduction | | | | | |
| Fruit and vegetables | | | | | |
| Fat intake | | | | | |
| Low salt diet | | | | | |
| Exercise | | | | | |
| Smoking cessation | | | | | |

## Finishing the Consultation

| | | | | | |
|---|---|---|---|---|---|
| Explore any difficulties in achieving goals, and offer a short term achievable aim | | | | | |
| Elicit patient concerns or questions | | | | | |
| Summarise back to the patient | | | | | |
| Arrange a follow up appointment (as necessary) or offer your contact details | | | | | |
| Thank patient and close consultation | | | | | |

## General Points

| | | | | | |
|---|---|---|---|---|---|
| Check patient understands regularly | | | | | |
| Maintain good eye contact and engage with patient | | | | | |
| Avoid medical jargon | | | | | |
| Polite to patient | | | | | |

Comm Skills

---

### What medications might a patient be started on after STEMI?

- Aspirin
- Clopidogrel or prasugrel or ticagrelor
- Statin
- Beta blocker
- ACE inhibitor

---

### When can the patient drive a car again? Does the DVLA need to be informed?

If successfully treated by coronary angioplasty, driving may recommence after one week, provided:

- No other URGENT revascularisation is planned (within four weeks from the acute event)
- Left ventricular ejection fraction (the fraction of blood pumped out of the left ventricle with each heartbeat) is at least 40% prior to hospital discharge
- There is no other disqualifying condition
- If not successfully treated by coronary angioplasty, driving may recommence after four weeks provided there is no other disqualifying condition
- The Driver and Vehicle Licensing Agency (DVLA) does not need to be notified

Comm Skills

> ## Name four complications associated with a myocardial infarction.
>
> - Cardiac arrhythmias (e.g. atrial fibrillation)
> - Pericarditis (and also Dressler's syndrome)
> - Cardiac valve pathology (e.g. mitral regurgitation)
> - Heart failure
> - Cardiogenic shock
> - Ventricular aneurysm
> - Reinfarction / angina
> - Depression

## Additional Questions to Consider

1 // When can they fly?

2 // When can they have sex?

3 // What are the side effects of ACE inhibitors?

4 // After having a CABG, what considerations need to be made when determining when the patient can go back to work?

5 // What are the risk factors for ischaemic heart disease, and which of these are modifiable?

# Station 9
## DEALING WITH AN AGITATED PATIENT

*Candidate Briefing: **Mr. Gates is a 65-year-old gentleman who has come to your clinic today. He is very angry because he was supposed to receive a staging CT scan for his bowel cancer over a month ago, and hasn't heard anything about it.***

*Patient Briefing: **Your name is Mr. Gates and you are 65 years old. You were diagnosed with bowel cancer over a month ago and were told that a CT scan would be arranged to determine whether the bowel cancer has spread to any other parts of the body and plan your subsequent treatment. You have come to the clinic today feeling very angry because you still have not received a date for your CT scan.***

When you initially meet the doctor you are very angry because the CT scan has not happened and that nobody has contacted you. You ask for an explanation why this has occurred. You tell the doctor that you were expecting to start treatment and are concerned that this delay will have given the cancer the opportunity to grow further. You want to know what the doctor is going to do. You ask the doctor when you will have your CT scan.

If the doctor is empathetic and able to answer your questions you will become less angry. If he agrees to arrange an urgent scan as soon as possible you will thank him and leave the consultation.

*If the doctor does not listen to you, interrupts you or criticizes you, you will become angrier and demand to speak to the consultant. Regardless, you want to make a formal complaint about what has happened.*

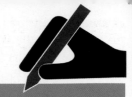

## Mark Scheme for Examiner

### Introduction

| | | | | | |
|---|---|---|---|---|---|
| Clean hands, introduce self, confirm patient identity | | | | | |
| Check identity of others in the room and confirm that the patient is happy for them to be present. Establish if patient would like anyone else present | | | | | |
| Establish current patient knowledge and concerns | | | | | |
| Allow the patient to vent their anger | | | | | |
| Ensure your own safety | | | | | |

### Positive Indicators

| | | | | | |
|---|---|---|---|---|---|
| Be focused on the patient | | | | | |
| Acknowledge the patient's concerns and explore origins of anger | | | | | |
| Summarise concerns back to patient | | | | | |
| Address the patient's concerns | | | | | |
| Formulate a realistic plan to address the overall problem | | | | | |

### Negative Indicators to Avoid

| | | | | | |
|---|---|---|---|---|---|
| Avoid attributing blame | | | | | |
| Avoid being defensive | | | | | |
| Avoid criticising the patient | | | | | |
| Avoid interrupting or patronising the patient | | | | | |
| Avoid giving no information | | | | | |

Comm Skills

## Dealing with a Difficult Patient

| | | | | | |
|---|---|---|---|---|---|
| Apologise again | | | | | |
| Offer if the patient would like to speak to the consultant | | | | | |
| Give clear boundaries to the patient if they are being aggressive | | | | | |

## Finishing the Consultation

| | | | | | |
|---|---|---|---|---|---|
| Ensure the patient has no further concerns or questions | | | | | |
| Summarise back to the patient the agreed plan | | | | | |
| Given information about the complaints procedure if still unhappy | | | | | |
| Arrange a follow up appointment (as necessary) or offer your contact details | | | | | |
| Thank patient and close consultation | | | | | |

## General Points

| | | | | | |
|---|---|---|---|---|---|
| Remain calm throughout | | | | | |
| Maintain good eye contact and engage with patient | | | | | |
| Polite to patient | | | | | |
| Validate the patient's feelings | | | | | |

Comm Skills

## What steps might you take if you knew that a scenario had the potential to escalate?

Preparation:
- Never turn your back on a potentially aggressive patient, and always sit nearest to the door, in case you have to make a quick escape
- Maintain your distance from the patient
- Notify someone else on the ward so that they can be aware that you might get into difficulties so that they can listen out for you
- In serious cases of aggression also warn security as they may need to be called in but it may not be suitable to bring anyone else into the room with you as this may aggravate the patient
- In cases on mental health wards it may also be suitable to bring a personal alarm into the room with you

*Remember 80% of communication is non-verbal:*
- Stay calm, speak slowly and politely
- Keep your voice at a conversational level
- Maintain eye contact
- Empathy can help. Show that you can understand the root of the patient's anger, e.g., "I know you feel angry about your long wait, but I'd like to try and help you with your chest pain"
- It is possible to regain control of a potentially volatile situation by asking the patient a few questions, e.g. who, what, why – to elicit their side of the story
- By identifying the cause of the aggression, you might be able to deal with it
- Document all conversations and patient concerns carefully
- Your own safety is paramount. If in doubt, get out

Comm Skills

**What are the different channels through which a patient could complain if they are not happy with the care they have received (up to two answers required)?**

- Local complaints manager
- Primary care trust complaints manager
- Patient advice liaison service
- General medical council

## Additional Questions to Consider

**1 //** How do you think the consultation went? What could have been done better?

**2 //** What do you think the patient's greatest underlying concern was in this case?

**3 //** What do you think the cause of the patient's anger was?

**4 //** What would you do if you noticed that a patient was prescribed and given the wrong medication on a ward round?

**5 //** The patient starts aggressively shouting and threatening you personally. What would you do next?

Comm Skills

# Station 10
# BREAKING BAD NEWS

*Scenario:* **Mrs. Gardner has come in to see you. You admitted her husband last week, who was suffering from a chest infection, on a long-term background of colorectal cancer. Despite antibiotic therapy, he is now rapidly deteriorating, and your consultant anticipates that Mr. Gardner has days, if not hours to live.**

*Relative Briefing:* **You name is Mrs. Gardner. You have come to see the doctor to speak about your husband who was admitted to hospital last week.**

You have been told so far that he is suffering from a chest infection. Your husband also has a background of colorectal cancer. You have been told that he has been having strong antibiotics through a drip but he appears to have been worsening rather than improving. He is coughing a lot and is short of breath on minimal exertion.

*Your main concern is that your husband is getting worse and not better. You are worried that he might not survive this infection. You report that your husband has always said that if he was to deteriorate from his cancer he would not have wanted to suffer. You have children that live four hours drive away and you want to know whether they should be called to see their father. You are also concerned that you gave this infection to your husband since you have recently had a chest infection as well, and feel guilty.*

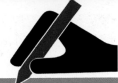

# Mark Scheme for Examiner

## Introduction

Clean hands, introduce self, confirm relative's identity

Check identity of others in the room and confirm that the relative is happy for them to be present, establish if relatives would like anyone else present

## Setting

Inform the examiner you would meet in a quite, private room and pass your bleep to another member of staff

## Perception

Elicit the relatives current understanding

Elicit current concerns and expectations

## Invitation

Establish what the relative would like to know

Set out a plan for what will happen in the consultation

## Knowledge

Use a warning shot to prepare the relative for bad news

Convey the bad news

Allow the relative time to take the news in

Answer any questions the relative may have

## Empathy

| | | | | | |
|---|---|---|---|---|---|
| Allow a period of silence | | | | | |
| Offer tissues if appropriate | | | | | |
| Allow the relative to express their emotions | | | | | |

## Strategy and Summary

| | | | | | |
|---|---|---|---|---|---|
| Offer reassurance or hope if possible | | | | | |
| Provide written information if available / appropriate | | | | | |
| Offer spiritual support e.g. refer to chaplain | | | | | |
| Arrange a follow up appointment (as necessary) or offer your contact details | | | | | |
| Close the consultation | | | | | |

## General Points

| | | | | | |
|---|---|---|---|---|---|
| Empathetic | | | | | |
| Avoid medical jargon | | | | | |
| Polite to relative | | | | | |
| Listens to relatives concerns | | | | | |

Comm Skills

## How do you think the consultation went?

- Reflects on what went well
- Reflects on what could have been done better
- Identified main concerns of the relative

## Do you know any recommended methods or guides on how you might break bad news to a patient?

- The SPIKES technique is an effective method to structure breaking bad news
- Setting (ensure appropriate setting)
- Perception (establish what the individual knows already)
- Invitation (establish what the patient would like to find out)
- Knowledge (impart information)
- Empathy (react appropriately to patient's emotions)
- Strategy and Summary (close conversation, arrange follow up, and outline on-going management plan)
- Another model to consider is the 10 step model (http://www.nursinghomes.cht.nhs.uk/fileadmin/Nursing/Docs/palliative/breaking_bad_news_guidelines.pdf)

## How much of this consultation do you think this relative will remember once they leave the room?

- It has been suggested that at best people remember about one third of any consultation
- In this stressful and emotionally charged scenario, it is likely to be less than this

Comm Skills

1 // What steps might you take prior to breaking bad news to any patient?

2 // What if the patient starts to cry while you are talking?

3 // You had a long talk with the patient yesterday, and today the nurse takes you aside to say the patient doesn't understand what is going on. What do you do?

4 // A family member has asked you not to tell their relative about their diagnosis of metastatic prostatic cancer. What are your options? What would you do?

5 // You witness another professional tell something to a patient in a really insensitive manner.
What would you do?

6 // What steps could you take to help the patient remember the important aspects of the consultation?

Comm Skills

# Chapter 5

# Practical Skills

# STATION 1
# INTERMEDIATE LIFE SUPPORT

*Candidate Briefing: You are on the medical wards and come across a patient collapsed on the floor. Approach the patient and perform resuscitation as necessary. Follow any instructions that are given by the examiners in this situation.*

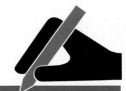

## Mark Scheme for Examiner

| BLS | | | | | |
|---|---|---|---|---|---|
| Look for danger | | | | | |
| Response, both ears | | | | | |
| Call for HELP | | | | | |
| Check for airway obstruction | | | | | |
| Head tilt. Chin lift | | | | | |
| Breathing – look and listen for 10 seconds | | | | | |
| Circulation – feel carotid for 10 seconds | | | | | |
| Tell help to call 2222 (location, cardiac arrest, adult / paediatric / pregnant) | | | | | |
| Chest compression x30, rate of 100 / min, to 1 / 3 depth of chest | | | | | |
| 2 breaths: ideally bag and valve mask connected to oxygen | | | | | |

*how to hold*

Practical

## ILS

| | | | | | |
|---|---|---|---|---|---|
| Ask helper to continue chest compressions and ventilation breaths | | | | | |
| Turn on defibrillator and place pads (whilst continuing CPR) | | | | | |
| Stop CPR to assess rhythm (all hands off patient) | | | | | |

## Shockable Rhythm

| | | | | | |
|---|---|---|---|---|---|
| Correctly identify rhythm: VF/VT | | | | | |
| Continue CPR | | | | | |
| Charge defibrillator to 150J (biphasic) 360J (monophasic) | | | | | |
| Command 'STAND CLEAR, OXYGEN AWAY' | | | | | |
| Double check rhythm again, then deliver shock 'SHOCKING' | | | | | |
| Resume CPR immediately | | | | | |
| CPR for two minutes then reassess | | | | | |
| Administer adrenaline and amioderone after the third shock, and give adrenaline every other shock | | | | | |

## Non Shockable Rhythm

| | | | | | |
|---|---|---|---|---|---|
| Correct identification of rhythm: PEA / asystole | | | | | |
| Adrenaline 1mg immediately | | | | | |
| CPR for 2 minutes then reassess | | | | | |
| Adrenaline every 3-5 minutes | | | | | |

## During the 2 Minute Cycles

| | | | | | |
|---|---|---|---|---|---|
| IV access | | | | | |
| ABG – (often femoral stab) for Hb, K+ and glucose | | | | | |
| Patient notes/clinical information for reversible causes i.e. 4H's and 4T's | | | | | |

Practical

## Post Resuscitation Care

| | | | | |
|---|---|---|---|---|
| Oxygen | | | | |
| Fluids | | | | |
| Full set of observations | | | | |
| ECG | | | | |
| Chest X-Ray | | | | |
| Inform HDU / ITU | | | | |

## Questions And Answers for Candidate

### What are the eight reversible causes of cardiac arrest?

- Hypovolaemia
- Hypotension
- Hypo / hyperkalaemia
- Hypothermia
- Thrombus
- Tamponade
- Tension pneumothorax
- Toxins

**In the cardiac arrest resuscitation cycle, what are the rhythms that are non-shockable?**

- Pulseless electrical activity, and asystole

**What are the three moves you might employ to open a compromised airway in an unconscious patient (when there is no suggestion of cervical spine injury)?**

- Head tilt
- Chin lift
- Jaw thrust

## Additional Questions to Consider

1 // What is the normal PR interval?

2 // What is the upper limit of QRS duration?

3 // Define hypothermia.

4 // Define bradycardia.

5 // Define wide complex QRS.

# STATION 2
# PHLEBOTOMY

*Candidate Briefing: Mr Federick is a 50-year-old man who is attending your clinic for an INR check, having recently been started on warfarin. Please explain to him what you are going to do, and then demonstrate how you would take blood on the mannequin.*

## Mark Scheme for Examiner

### Introduction and General Preparation

| | | | | | |
|---|---|---|---|---|---|
| Introduce self (wash hands before touching patient) | | | | | |
| Identify patient (5 points of ID) | | | | | |
| Explain procedure and identify concerns e.g. needlephobia | | | | | |
| Chose correct site (patient preference, any pain, medical / surgical issues) | | | | | |
| Allergies | | | | | |
| Position patient comfortably | | | | | |

### Procedure Preparation

| | | | | | |
|---|---|---|---|---|---|
| Decontaminate hands | | | | | |
| Clean tray according to local policy | | | | | |
| Gather all equipment (including checking expiry dates) | | | | | |
| Assemble equipment using non touch technique (needle to vacutainer) | | | | | |

Practical

## Drawing Blood

| | | | | | |
|---|---|---|---|---|---|
| Apply single use disposable apron | | | | | |
| Apply disposable tourniquet | | | | | |
| Select appropriate vein and loosen tourniquet | | | | | |
| Clean hands and apply gloves | | | | | |
| Clean site for 30 seconds | | | | | |
| Warn patient | | | | | |
| Puncture vein and withdraw blood | | | | | |
| Remove tourniquet | | | | | |
| Remove needle and apply pressure with gauze | | | | | |
| Immediately dispose of sharps | | | | | |
| Apply a sterile dressing | | | | | |
| Label the bottles at the bedside | | | | | |
| Tell patient to inform staff if site becomes painful or continues to bleed; can remove dressing after a few hours | | | | | |

## Finishing

| | | | | |
|---|---|---|---|---|
| Dispose of equipment | | | | |
| Clean tray | | | | |
| Wash hands | | | | |

## General Points

| | | | | |
|---|---|---|---|---|
| Continuous talking through the procedure to patient | | | | |
| Dispose of all sharp needles immediately | | | | |
| Avoided patient contamination (i.e. non touch technique NTT followed throughout) | | | | |

Practical

## What is the order of draw for FBC, U&Es, and clotting?

1. Clotting
2. U&Es
3. FBC

## Give some examples of what might cause hyperkalaemia.

- Renal failure
- Drugs (e.g. ACE inhibitors, potassium sparing diuretics)
- Addisons disease
- Aldosterone deficiency
- Metabolic acidosis
- Excessive intake
- Haemolysis (e.g. during venepuncture)

## What additives are found in the different blood tubes?

- Full Blood Count: EDTA
- Clotting studies: citrate
- Plasma analysis: lithium heparin (or sodium heparin)
- Glucose: potassium oxalate and sodium fluoride
- Serum tube: no additive: because you want the blood to clot and centrifuge the serum

Practical

**1 //**   What is D-dimer and what does it signify?

**2 //**   Name some acute phase substances commonly tested.

**3 //**   What is meant by left shift or right shift on a blood film?

**4 //**   How is calcium affected by application of a tourniquet to take a blood sample?

**5 //**   What does the APTT reflect?

**6 //**   What is adjusted calcium or corrected calcium, and how is it calculated?

Practical

# STATION 3
# INTRAVENOUS CANNULATION

*Candidate Briefing: Mrs Jones has been diagnosed with small bowel obstruction. She requires intravenous fluids. Please obtain consent for this and then, on the mannequin provided, demonstrate how to insert an intravenous cannula.*

## Mark Scheme for Examiner

## Introduction and General Preparation

| | | | | | |
|---|---|---|---|---|---|
| Introduce self (wash hands before touching patient) | | | | | |
| Identify patient (5 points of ID) | | | | | |
| Explain procedure | | | | | |
| Chose correct site (patient preference, any pain, medical / surgical issues) | | | | | |
| Allergies | | | | | |
| Position patient comfortably | | | | | |
| Gather all equipment (including checking expiration dates) | | | | | |
| Ask patient to wash hands / arms if possible | | | | | |

## Prepare Intravenous Extension Set

| | | | | | |
|---|---|---|---|---|---|
| Wash hands | | | | | |
| Clean tray | | | | | |
| Wash hands and put on non-sterile gloves | | | | | |
| Draw up saline immediately discarding needle | | | | | |
| Flush intravenous extension set (keeping it in packet, and clamping the line) | | | | | |

Practical

## Prepare Flush and Cannula

| | | | | | |
|---|---|---|---|---|---|
| Draw up saline immediately discarding needle | | | | | |
| Attach syringe to second sheathed needle (or sterile cap) for storage | | | | | |
| Open all packaging for cannula so can be accessed later | | | | | |
| Remove gloves and wash hands | | | | | |

## Insert Cannula

| | | | | | |
|---|---|---|---|---|---|
| Apply apron | | | | | |
| Position arm | | | | | |
| Apply tourniquet, select vein, then loosen tourniquet | | | | | |
| Wash hands | | | | | |
| Non sterile gloves on | | | | | |
| Retighten tourniquet | | | | | |
| Clean site (30 seconds) and air dry (30 seconds) | | | | | |
| Insert cannula (without palpating aseptic area) | | | | | |
| Release tourniquet | | | | | |
| Remove needle (whilst occluding vein) and immediately dispose to sharps bin | | | | | |
| Attach intravenous extension set, and then clean any leakage of blood | | | | | |
| Apply sterile dressing (pre labeled with date and time) | | | | | |

## Flush the Cannula

| | | | | | |
|---|---|---|---|---|---|
| Clean end of intravenous extension set (30 seconds) and air dry (30 seconds) | | | | | |
| Attach preprepared flush, and flush 1ml at a time, explaining to patient what they might feel | | | | | |
| Close clip whilst last ml is being flushed, and remove syringe | | | | | |

## Finishing

| | | | | |
|---|---|---|---|---|
| Clean tray | | | | |
| Dispose of equipment (clinical waste bin) | | | | |
| Remove gloves | | | | |
| Wash hands | | | | |
| Place 'cannula insertion record' in notes | | | | |
| Explain to patient what to watch out for | | | | |

## General Points

| | | | | |
|---|---|---|---|---|
| Continuous talking through the procedure to patient | | | | |
| Dispose of all sharps immediately | | | | |
| Avoided patient contamination (i.e. non touch technique NTT followed throughout) | | | | |

## Setting up a Giving Set

| | | | | |
|---|---|---|---|---|
| Wash hands and put on non sterile gloves | | | | |
| Check bag of fluid with examiner | | | | |
| Is it the same fluid and quantity as what is prescribed on the fluid chart? | | | | |
| Are any additives required? | | | | |
| Is it in date? | | | | |
| Check that there is no sediment floating in the fluid bag | | | | |
| Check that the bag has not leaked into the packaging | | | | |
| Write down the batch number on the chart | | | | |
| Remove from outer casing | | | | |
| Remove giving set from the bag and close the tap | | | | |
| Remove the cap from the fluid bag and attach it to the giving set | | | | |
| Place bag on stand | | | | |

| Squeeze the chamber at the top of the giving set until it is filled halfway with fluid | | | | | |
|---|---|---|---|---|---|
| **SLOWLY** open the tap of the giving set so that fluid flows down the line | | | | | |
| Attach line to cannula | | | | | |
| Remove gloves | | | | | |
| Dispose of equipment in clinical waste bin | | | | | |
| Wash hands | | | | | |
| Document date and time of start of fluid infusion | | | | | |

## Questions And Answers for Candidate

Practical

### What is the order of sizes of cannulas available on an adult medical ward?

- Brown / Orange (14G): large infusion / emergency
- Grey (16G): rapid infusion / obstetrics
- White / Green (18G): blood transfusion / fluid infusion / certain medications e.g. amiodarone
- Pink (20G): fluids / bolus medication
- Blue (22G): fluids / bolus medication

### What is the smallest gauge cannula recommended for blood transfusion?

- 20 gauge can be used, although 18 gauge is preferred

> **What factor is the most critical determinant of flow rate through a cannula?**

- The radius of the cannula bore; flow rate is proportional to the radius to the power of 4 (Note: diameter is also an acceptable answer to this question)

## Additional Questions to Consider

**1 //** What is the current maximum duration recommended for peripheral cannula to remain in situ, to avoid or reduce the incidence of Staph aureus bacteraemia?

**2 //** What veins are considered "central" in terms of cannulation?

**3 //** What are the complications of intravenous cannulation?

**4 //** Apart from anatomical location, what else might suggest to you that you had accidentally cannulated an artery instead of a vein?

**5 //** In an emergency, if you cannot gain intravenous access, what other routes are acceptable for drug delivery?

Practical

# STATION 4
# MALE URETHRAL CATHETERISATION

*Candidate Briefing: Mr Miller has lower abdominal pain and has been sent to the accident and emergency department by his GP. You diagnose acute urinary retention. Mr Miller requires a urethral catheter. Having already obtained his consent, demonstrate this procedure on the mannequin provided.*

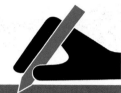

## Mark Scheme for Examiner

### Introduction and General Preparation

| | | | | | |
|---|---|---|---|---|---|
| Introduce self (wash hands before touching patient) | | | | | |
| Identify patient (5 points of ID) | | | | | |
| Explain procedure | | | | | |
| Position patient and provide blanket to maintain dignity | | | | | |
| Ask for chaperone/assistant | | | | | |
| Select appropriate catheter | | | | | |

### Procedure Preparation

| | | | | | |
|---|---|---|---|---|---|
| Decontaminate hands | | | | | |
| Clean tray according to local policy | | | | | |
| Gather all equipment (including checking expiry dates) | | | | | |
| Open catheterization pack (using non touch technique: NTT) | | | | | |
| Using NTT open outer packaging and drop Instillagel®, gloves and catheter onto aseptic field | | | | | |
| Open the packaging of the catheter bag | | | | | |
| If not provided with catheter set, draw up 10ml sterile water using green needle to use to inflate catheter balloon later on (dispose of sharps appropriately) | | | | | |

## Prepare the Patient

| | | | | | |
|---|---|---|---|---|---|
| Expose umbilicus to knees. Ensure patient dignity (shut curtains / door) provide blanket | | | | | |
| Wash hands | | | | | |
| Apply apron and sterile gloves | | | | | |
| Lay sterile drape with central hole for penis | | | | | |

## Asepsis and Anesthesia

| | | | | | |
|---|---|---|---|---|---|
| Ask assistant to empty sterile water into plastic pot | | | | | |
| Hold penis with non dominant hand, retract prepuce and clean with cotton wool swabs soaked in sterile water | | | | | |
| Dispose of swabs outside of aseptic field | | | | | |
| Warn patient and administer Instillagel®; wait 2 minutes to take effect | | | | | |
| Remove gloves, put on second pair of sterile gloves | | | | | |

## Inserting the Catheter

| | | | | | |
|---|---|---|---|---|---|
| Place disposable dish between legs to catch urine | | | | | |
| Hold penis in non dominant hand and apply upward traction | | | | | |
| Introduce catheter to urethral meatus until urine passes or significant resistance / pain | | | | | |
| Inflate balloon with 10mls of sterile water from pre filled syringe; ask if painful and *STOP* if patient does complain of pain | | | | | |
| Connect catheter to catheter bag or attach to leg bag if present | | | | | |
| Replace the prepuce | | | | | |
| Clean the patient remove drape and recover patient | | | | | |
| Dispose of waste and gloves, then wash hands | | | | | |
| Clean trolley then wash hands | | | | | |

| Tell to inform staff if becomes painful | | | | | |
| Document insertion in patient's medical notes | | | | | |

## General Points

| Continuous talking through the procedure to patient | | | | | |
| Dispose of all sharp needles immediately | | | | | |
| Avoided patient contamination (i.e. non touch technique NTT followed throughout) | | | | | |

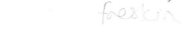

foreskin

## Questions And Answers for Candidate

### What are the risks of urethral catheterization (name 3)?

- Trauma (false passage, damage to urethral sphincters)
- Infection
- Bladder spasm
- Paraphimosis (failure to replace prepuce)

### What types of urinary catheter are commonly available?

- A foley catheter
- Silastic catheter (which tends to be used for a longer term)
- Suprapubic catheter

## Additional Questions to Consider

**1 //**  What is an atonic bladder?

**2 //**  What do you need to document in the notes after inserting a catheter?

**3 //**  What is the system for describing catheter sizes?

**4 //**  What fluid should you fill a catheter balloon with? (or what should you NOT fill it with?)

**5 //**  What would you do if you met significant resistance when blowing up the catheter balloon?

Practical

# STATION 5
# URINALYSIS

*Candidate Briefing: Mrs Manpreet is a 35 year-old female who present to your clinic with abdominal pain and vomiting. She has been going to the toilet more often than normal and is concerned that her urine is foul-smelling. She has bought a urine sample with her. Please perform a urine dipstick and discuss the results with her.*

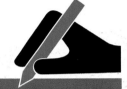

## Mark Scheme for Examiner

### Obtaining the Urine Sample (if not provided)

| | | | | | |
|---|---|---|---|---|---|
| Provide patient with sterile urine pot | | | | | |
| Ask for a mid stream sample | | | | | |
| Explain how to collect a midstream sample | | | | | |

### Urine Dipstick

| | | | | | |
|---|---|---|---|---|---|
| Wash hands | | | | | |
| Apply gloves and apron | | | | | |
| Inspect sample | | | | | |
| Remove cap – comment on any odour | | | | | |
| Check expiry date on dipstick container, and remove a single dipstick | | | | | |
| Dip in the urine ensuring all rectangles submerged for 2-3 seconds | | | | | |
| Leave dipstick horizontal to dry and develop for 1 minute | | | | | |
| Use colour chart on dipstick box to interpret results | | | | | |

## Interpretation

Comment on: blood, ketones, nitrites, protein, glucose, specific gravity, pH

## Questions And Answers for Candidate

### Which two results are commonly positive in an uncomplicated UTI?

- Nitrites and leukocytes (most important answers)
- pH (alkaline if proteus), may also get blood or protein

### When might you get a false-positive glucose test on urine dip?

- The presence of other substances in the urine can interfere with the test strips and give a false positive
- Examples include aspirin, penicillin, isoniazid, vitamin c, and cephalosporins

### What does the presence of red cell casts on light microscopy suggest?

- Glomerulonephritis

Practical

1 // Name some causes of proteinuria.

2 // What is microalbuminuria, and how is it detected?

3 // What is the significance of ketones on urine dipstick?

4 // What bacteria are commonly associated with staghorn calculi?

5 // What else can be tested for on a urine dipstick?

# STATION 6
# ECG INTERPRETATION

*Candidate Briefing: Mr Fredrickson (DOB 7/3/1950) has been having severe chest pain for two hours. He is a smoker, and is known to suffer from diabetes. An ECG had been performed. Please assess the ECG below, and present your findings.*

Taken on 28/2/2013 at 1915
Mr Fredrickson (DOB 7/3/1950)
Paper speed: 25mm/second (standard)
Calibration: 10mm/mV (standard)

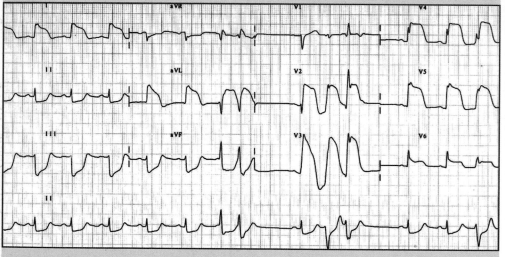

ECG 1, (Image 5 Chapter 5, Station 6: Unofficial Guide to Passing OSCEs 3rd Edition)

The Unofficial Guide to Passing OSCEs: *Candidate Briefings, Patient Briefings and Mark Schemes*

## Additional ECGs for practice (same paper speed and calibration)

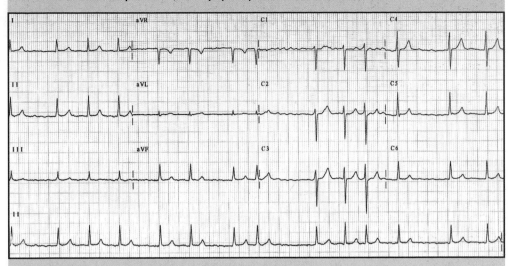

ECG 2: (Image 2 Chapter 5, Station 6: Unofficial Guide to Passing OSCEs 3rd Edition)

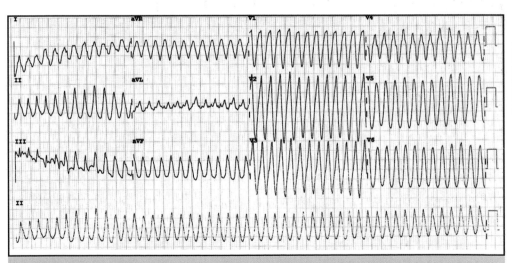

ECG 3: (Image 7 Chapter 5, Station 6: Unofficial Guide to Passing OSCEs 3rd Edition)

# Mark Scheme for Examiner

## General

| | | | | | |
|---|---|---|---|---|---|
| Time and date of ECG | | | | | |
| Patient details | | | | | |
| Calibration | | | | | |
| Paper speed | | | | | |
| Heart rate | | | | | |
| Rhythms | | | | | |
| Cardiac axis | | | | | |

## Morphology (comment on the following)

| | | | | | |
|---|---|---|---|---|---|
| P waves (morphology and relation to QRS complexes) | | | | | |
| PR interval | | | | | |
| QRS complex (wide or narrow) | | | | | |
| ST segment (elevated or depressed) | | | | | |
| T waves (inversion, flattening, biphasic, tented) | | | | | |
| Q wave (pathological or non pathological) | | | | | |
| QT interval | | | | | |
| Present findings, with diagnosis | | | | | |

Practical

**Findings on ECG 1:**
'The heart rate is 82 bpm, the rhythm is regular. The axis is within normal limits. P waves are present, PR interval is normal, and QRS complexes are narrow. There is massive ST elevation, up to 16mm, in leads I, AVL, V2-6, and T wave inversion in lead aVL. There is ST reciprocal depression in leads II, III and aVF. 4 ectopics are also present. The QT interval is normal. In summary, this ECG is consistent with an anterolateral ST elevation myocardial infarction, with reciprocal inferior ST depression.'

**Findings on ECG 2:**
'The heart rate is 84 bpm, the rhythm is irregularly irregular. The axis is within normal limits. No P waves are present. QRS complexes are narrow, and there are no ST or T wave changes. The QT interval is normal. In summary, this ECG is consistent with atrial fibrillation.'

**Findings on ECG 3:**
'The heart rate is 300 bpm, the rhythm is regular. The axis is within normal limits. P waves are not clearly visible. QRS complexes are wide. ST segment and T wave changes cannot be seen. In summary, this ECG is consistent with a broad complex tachycardia (either ventricular tachycardia or supraventicular tachycardia with bundle branch block). QT interval is not possible to assess. My priority is to check if the patient is conscious and has an output.'

---

**What would be your immediate management of patient with chest pain and a suspected anterolateral ST elevation acute coronary syndrome?**

- Resuscitate the patient using an ABCDE approach
- Morphine 5-10mg IV + Metoclopramide 10mg IV
- High flow oxygen
- Nitrates – GTN 2 puffs sublingual
- Asprin 300mg
- Clopidogrel or prasugrel or ticagrelor
- IV access
- Bloods: FBC, U&E, Glucose, Lipids, Cardiac enzymes
- Consider immediate percutaneous coronary intervention, or thrombolysis if PCI not available within the recommended timeframe

---

**What is the voltage criteria for left ventricular hypertrophy?**

- The height of the 'S' wave in V1 or V2 plus the size of the 'R' wave in V5 or V6 is determined by counting the number of small squares. If the sum of these two is greater than 40, then LVH is suggested or suspected (not confirmed)

---

**What is meant by reciprocal changes, for example in an anterior STEMI?**

- This is where you have ST elevation in one territory – in this case, the anterior aspect, and ST depression in another – in this case it would be the inferior leads

## Which leads look at each aspect of the heart?

- Anterior – V1 – V4
- Lateral – I, aVL, V5 – V6
- Inferior – II, III, aVF
- Posterior – not directly visualised

You suspect a posterior MI by looking at the anterior leads V1-V3 and see changes that are inverted (or reciprocal). You need to extend the chest leads around the back to see the posterior surface.

## Additional Questions to Consider

**1 //** Explain how you determine the cardiac axis.

**2 //** Give some examples of regularly irregular rhythms on an ECG.

**3 //** Name some drugs used for inotropic support.

**4 //** What is pre-excitation and how does it look on an ECG?

**5 //** List some causes of RBBB and LBBB.

Practical

# STATION 7
# FUNDOSCOPY

*Candidate Briefing: Mr Wilson is a 55-year-old man with diabetes. Please examine his fundi. His pupils have already been dilated. Sketch your findings on the sheet provided.*

IMAGE 1: (Fig 5.3 Chapter 5, Station 7: Unofficial Guide to Passing OSCEs)

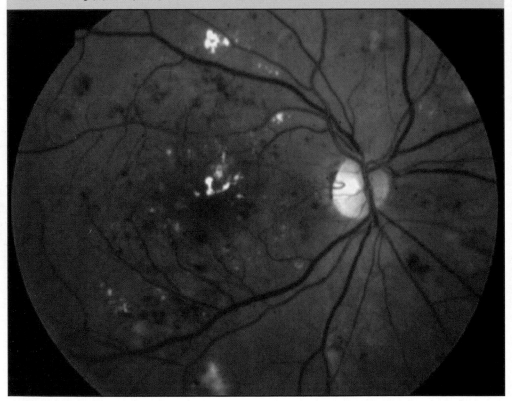

Additional Images to Practice:
(follow on the next page)

**IMAGE 2: (Fig 5.5 Chapter 5, Station 7: Unofficial Guide to Passing OSCEs)**

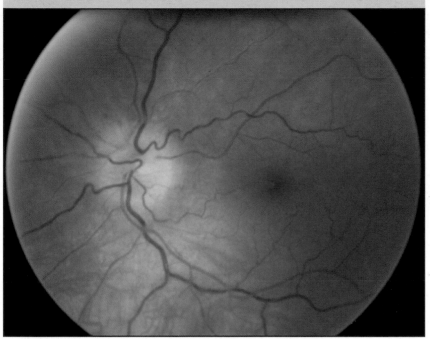

**IMAGE 3 (Fig 6 Chapter 5, Station 7: Unofficial Guide to Passing OSCEs)**

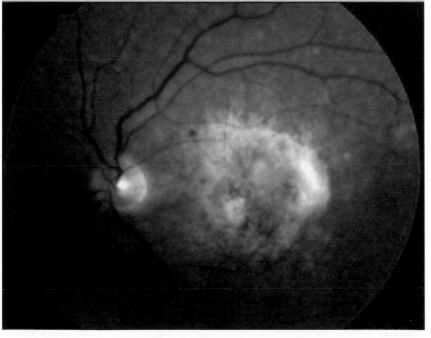

## Introduction and General Preparation

| | | | | | |
|---|---|---|---|---|---|
| Introduce self (wash hands before touching patient) | | | | | |
| Seek permission | | | | | |
| Explain procedure: warn will be close to face | | | | | |

## Positioning and Technique

| | | | | | |
|---|---|---|---|---|---|
| Darken room | | | | | |
| Ensure pupil dilated (e.g. using tropicamide) | | | | | |
| Correct set up and adjustment of ophthalmoscope | | | | | |
| Examine the right eye with your right eye (scope in right hand) and visa versa | | | | | |

## Examination Sequence

| | | | | | |
|---|---|---|---|---|---|
| Elicit red reflex (At 30cm and 45 degree angle to nose) | | | | | |
| Examine optic disc | | | | | |
| Look for abnormalities in the macula | | | | | |
| Examine the four major vessels arcs out to the periphery, and look for retinal/vessel abnormalities in each quadrant | | | | | |
| Report your findings (see below) | | | | | |

---

*Findings on Image 1:*
'Multiple dot and blot haemorrhages are scattered throughout the retina. There are hard exudates in the superior field, and a cotton wool spot in the inferior field. The disc looks healthy, with no new vessels visible. These changes would be consistent with severe non-proliferative diabetic retinopathy. There are also hard exudates superior to the macula indicating diabetic maculopathy'

**Findings on Image 2:**
'The optic disc is pale with blurred margin, indicating a swollen disc.
If that patient has raised intracranial pressure this would be consistent
with papilloedema. I would also consider other causes such as optic neuritis'

**Findings on Image 3:**
'There is a pale area around the macula, with some hyperpigmented areas. There
are some soft drusen. I cannot see any areas of haemorrhage. This would be
consistent with dry age-related macular degeneration'

## Questions And Answers for Candidate

Practical

### What finding would you expect in non-proliferative diabetic retinopathy?

- Microaneurysms
- 'Dot and blot' haemorrhages
- Hard exudates
- Cotton wool spots

### What is laser photocoagulation and how does it treat diabetic retinopathy?

- The aim is to reduce the oxygen demand of the retina and thereby control, reduce or reverse neovascularisation
- Typically about 2000 low intensity burns are created in the periphery

## What are the stages seen in hypertensive retinopathy?

- Grade 1 = Silver wiring
- Grade 2 = Grade 1 plus AV nipping
- Grade 3 = Grade 2 plus cotton wool spots & flame haemorrhages
- Grade 4 = Grade 3 plus papilloedema

## ? Additional Questions to Consider

1 // Name some causes of a "cherry red spot".

2 // What is a cataract, and name some risk factors for its development?

3 // What is the red reflex? Why do we look for it in child surveillance?

4 // What does uveitis look like, and name a cause?

5 // Define the terms: strabismus, amblyopia, arcus, and pterygium.

# STATION 8
# DEATH CERTIFICATION

*Candidate Briefing: You are working on the stroke unit (at Hope Hospital, Whitby Road, London OG1 P02), and are called by the nursing staff to see an 81 year old patient (Jonathon Benjamin Morgue) that has just passed away. You are asked to pronounce them dead and to write a death certificate.*

*The cause of death is a cerebrovascular accident which happened 2 days ago. It was felt to be secondary to atrial fibrillation, which was diagnosed 1 year 5 months ago. The patient also suffered a myocardial infarction 11 years ago, and was diagnosed with COPD 16 years ago. There is a clear cause of death, and there are no other concerns with regard to informing the coroner. You clerked the patient on admission.*

*The patient was found dead by the nursing staff at 01am on 28/1/13, and you verify the death at 01:43. You're consultant is Dr. Raj Patel.*

*A blank death certificate is provided for you.* (on the following page)

Practical

# Medical certificate of cause of death

## Name of deceased

| Date of death | Day | Month | Year | | | | Time of death | Hour | Min |
|---|---|---|---|---|---|---|---|---|---|

Place of death

## Cause of death

I hereby certify that to the best of my knowledge and belief, the cause of death was as stated below:

Approximate interval between onset and death

| | | Years | Months | Days |
|---|---|---|---|---|

1. Disease or condition directly leading to death — a.)

**Antecedent causes**
Morbid conditions, if any, giving rise to above cause, stating the underlying condition last

b.)

c.)

d.)

2. Other significant conditions contributing to the death, but not related to the disease or condition causing it

Please tick the relevant box

**Post mortem**

PM1 ☐ Post mortem has been done and information is included above

PM2 ☐ Post mortem information may be available later

PM3 ☐ No post mortem is being done

**Procurator fiscal/Coroner**

PF ☐ This death has been reported to the procurator fiscal/coroner

**Attendance on deceased**

A1 ☐ I was in attendance upon the deceased during last illness

A2 ☐ I was not in attendance upon the deceased during last illness: the doctor who was is unable to provide the certificate

A3 ☐ No doctor was in attendance on the deceased

Signature
Name in
BLOCK CAPITALS
Official address

Date: _____

**For a death in hospital**
Name of the consultant
responsible

---

**Counterfoil – Medical certificate of cause of death**

Name of deceased
Date of death
Place of death

| Please circle as appropriate | | | | |
|---|---|---|---|---|
| Post mortem | PM1 | PM2 | PM3 | |
| Procurator fiscal/Coroner | PF | | | |
| Attendance on decreased | A1 | A2 | A3 | |

Cause of death
I (a)
(b)
(c)
(d)
II

Date of certificate

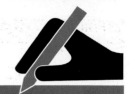

## Mark Scheme for Examiner

### Verification of Death

| | | | | | |
|---|---|---|---|---|---|
| If family present explain what you are going to do | | | | | |
| Check for response to painful stimuli (sternal rub) | | | | | |
| Feel for carotid pulse – 1 minute | | | | | |

### Positioning and Technique

| | | | | | |
|---|---|---|---|---|---|
| Auscultate for breath sounds – 1 minute | | | | | |
| Auscultate for heart sounds – 1 minute | | | | | |
| Check pupils for dilation and responsiveness to light | | | | | |
| Leave body in dignified state (cover up to neck in sheet) | | | | | |
| Document examination together with time and date of verification in the patients medical notes | | | | | |

### Writing a Death Certificate

| | | | | | |
|---|---|---|---|---|---|
| Block capitals and black ink used, no abbreviations used | | | | | |
| Patients full name, date of death and time of death as pronounced by doctor, place of death | | | | | |
| Select appropriate option regarding post-mortem | | | | | |
| Select appropriate option with regard to whether the doctor attended / another medical profession attended the deceased during their last illness | | | | | |
| Appropriate cause of death part one, including duration of disease(s) | | | | | |
| Appropriate significant co-morbidites in part two, including duration of disease(s) | | | | | |
| Your details (name, signature, medical qualification) | | | | | |
| Name of consultant in charge | | | | | |

Practical

# Medical certificate of cause of death

**Name of deceased** MR. JONATHON BENJAMIN MORGUE

| Date of death | Day | | Month | | Year | | | Time of death | Hour | | Min | |
|---|---|---|---|---|---|---|---|---|---|---|---|---|
| | 2 | 8 | 0 | 1 | 2 | 0 | 1 3 | | 0 | 1 | 4 | 3 |

**Place of death** STROKE UNIT, HOPE HOSPITAL WHITBY ROAD, LONDON, OG1 PO2

## Cause of death

I hereby certify that to the best of my knowledge and belief, the cause of death was as stated below:

**Approximate interval between onset and death**

| | | Years | Months | Days |
|---|---|---|---|---|
| 1. Disease or condition directly leading to death | a.) CEREBROVASCULAR ACCIDENT | | | 2 |
| **Antecedent causes** Morbid conditions, if any, | b.) ATRIAL FIBRILLATION | 1 | 5 | |
| giving rise to above cause, | c.) | | | |
| stating the underlying condition last | d.) | | | |

| | | | | |
|---|---|---|---|---|
| 2. Other significant conditions contributing to the | MYOCARDIAL INFARCTION | 11 | | |
| death, but not related to the disease or condition causing it | CHRONIC OBSTRUCTIVE PULMONARY DISEASE | 16 | | |

Please tick the relevant box

**Post mortem**

PM1 ☐ Post mortem has been done and information is included above

PM2 ☐ Post mortem information may be available later

PM3 ☑ No post mortem is being done

**Procurator fiscal/Coroner**

PF ☐ This death has been reported to the procurator fiscal/coroner

**Attendance on deceased**

A1 ☑ I was in attendance upon the deceased during last illness

A2 ☐ I was not in attendance upon the deceased during last illness: the doctor who was is unable to provide the certificate

A3 ☐ No doctor was in attendance on the deceased

| | |
|---|---|
| Signature | **Date:** 28.01.2013 |
| Name in | **For a death in hospital** |
| BLOCK CAPITALS DR KATE JONES | Name of the consultant |
| Official address STROKE UNIT, HOPE HOSPITAL, WHITBY ROAD, LONDON OG1 PO2 | responsible DR RAJ PATEL |

- - - - - - - - - - - - - - - - - - - - - - - - - - - - - - - - - - - - - - - - - - - - - - - - - - - -

**Counterfoil – Medical certificate of cause of death**

**Name of deceased** MR. JONATHON BENJAMIN MORGUE

**Date of death** 28.01.2013

**Place of death** STROKE UNIT, HOPE HOSPITAL, WHITBY ROAD, LONDON, OG1 PO2

Please circle as appropriate

| Post mortem | PM1 | PM2 | (PM3) |
|---|---|---|---|
| Procurator fiscal/Coroner | PF | | |
| Attendance on decreased | (A1) | A2 | A3 |

**Cause of death**

I (a) CEREBROVASCULAR ACCIDENT

(b) ATRIAL FIBRILLATION

(c)

(d)

II MYOCARDIAL INFARCTION

CHRONIC OBSTRUCTIVE PULMONARY DISEASE

**Date of certificate** 28.01.2013

Practical

### Give three examples of when a death might be reported to a coroner.

- Any uncertified death
- Any death that is sudden and unexpected, or that is violent, suspicious or unexplained
- Any death that results from an accident at work, involving a vehicle, or burns, scalds, fire, explosives or similar
- Due to poisioning, including overdose
- Due to industrial disease
- Where circumstances suggest suicide
- Indications of a medical mishap
- Following abortion
- Any death due to a fault or neglect on the behalf of another person or organisation
- Death occurring whilst in custody
- Death as a result of food poisoning or notifiable infectious disease
- Any death of a foster child

Practical

### Who can issue a death certificate?

- A registered medical practitioner or a coroner (or Procurator Fiscal in Scotland)

### Before cremation, what must be removed?

- Pacemakers or any kind of radioactive implant

**1** // Why is it important to check a patient's employment history in some cases?

**2** // What criteria must the doctor who completes the 2nd part of the cremation form meet in order to be allowed to fill it in?

**3** // When is the time of death, that which the patient is found dead by the nursing staff, or that which the patient is pronounced dead by the doctor?

**4** // What would you do if you were asked to pronounce a death in the middle of the night, but were not sure what the cause of death was?

**5** // The nurse calls you in the middle of the night as the on-call doctor to come and certify a death. What does the phrase 'certify a death' mean?

# STATION 9
# INSTRUMENTS

*Candidate Briefing: On this table there are a number of instruments.
Please take one and tell me what you know about it.*

(INSTRUMENT 1 (top left), 2 (top right), 3 (bottom left), 4 (bottom right). Images taken from Chapter 5, Station 9: Unofficial Guide to Passing OSCEs)

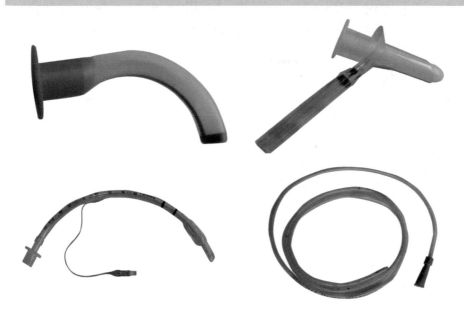

## Mark Scheme for Examiner

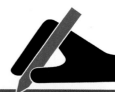

| Instruments | | | | | | |
|---|---|---|---|---|---|---|
| Name and type of instrument accurately described | | | | | | |
| Indication for use clearly given | | | | | | |
| Description of how to use the instrument given | | | | | | |
| Complications described of its use: at least three given | | | | | | |

**Findings for Instrument 1:**

1) 'This is an oropharyngeal (Guedel) airway; it is an example of a non-definitive airway adjunct.'

2) 'I have seen this being used in a patient with an impaired conscious level, and an unprotected airway presenting to accident and emergency.'

3) 'It is sized by measuring the distance from the incisors to the angle of the jaw. It is then introduced to the oral cavity, with the spout pointing superiorly and rotated 180 as it descends past the hard palate, entering the oropharynx. This approach reduces the risk of pushing the tongue backwards.'

4) 'Complications include trauma to the oropharynx, upper airway obstruction and stimulation of vomiting.'

**Findings for Instrument 2:**

1) 'This is a disposable proctoscope.'

2) 'I have seen this being used in an outpatient clinic to visualise and treat haemorrhoids.'

3) 'The patient is positioned in the left lateral position with their buttocks to the edge of the examination couch. The anus and perineum is inspected for evidence of fissures, fistula, prolapsed haemorrhoids or skin tags. A digital rectal examination is then performed. The proctoscope is connected to a non-disposable light source and then lubricated before being inserted slowly under direct vision. The obturator is removed and rectum visualised for diagnostic and therapeutic intervention.'

4) 'Complications include pain, perforation of the rectum, bleeding and damage to the anal sphincter.'

**Findings for Instrument 3:**

1) 'This is a cuffed endotracheal tube, it is an example of a definitive airway.'

2) 'I have seen this being used in intensive care for the ventilation of an unconscious patient.'

3) 'It is inserted by a trained health professional in a controlled environment. I have seen it inserted using direct laryngoscopy to identify the glottis. After insertion, a balloon cuff is inflated to secure it in place and to reduce the risk of aspirate entering the respiratory tract.'

4) 'Complications include those associated with the tube (subglottic stenosis, vocal cord paralysis) and those associated with the intubation procedure (misplacement, dental trauma, intubation of oesophagus, pulmonary aspiration).'

*Findings for Instrument 4:*

1) 'This is a Ryles nasogastric tube, of which there are two types: fine and wide-bore.'

2) 'I have seen fine-bore tubes being used to provide enteric feeding and witnessed wide-bore tubes used to provide gastric decompression in bowel obstruction.'

3) 'The lower 10cm is lubricated. It is then inserted into the patent nostril of an upright patient. It is advanced in a horizontal plane along the base of the nasal cavity. When it reaches the posterior pharynx, the patient is asked to swallow water through a straw, thereby introducing the tip into the oesophagus. The nasogastric tube is inserted to the 40cm mark and correct positioning is confirmed with pH aspirate (pH<4) and chest X-ray.'

4) 'Complications include damage to the nasal turbinates and oesophageal perforation. Care should be taken not to place the tube in the trachea.'

## Additional Questions to Consider

The same four questions (applied in this chapter) can be used for any instrument / medical equipment e.g. foley catheter, central line, chest drain.

# STATION 10
# SUTURING

*Candidate Briefing: Mr Harrison, 27, has presented to A&E with a simple laceration to his forearm. Please suture the wound together using simple interrupted sutures.*

## Mark Scheme for Examiner

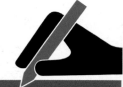

### Introduction and General Preparation

| | | | | | |
|---|---|---|---|---|---|
| Introduce self (wash hands before touching patient) | | | | | |
| Identify patient | | | | | |
| Explain procedure | | | | | |
| Assess the wound i.e. does it require senior involvement or plastic surgery referral | | | | | |
| Allergies | | | | | |
| Gather all appropriate equipment | | | | | |

### Wound Preparation

| | | | | | |
|---|---|---|---|---|---|
| Wash hands, apply sterile gloves | | | | | |
| Assemble equipment maintaining asepsis | | | | | |
| Remove visible debris with forceps | | | | | |
| Administer local anesthetic (pre cleaning) | | | | | |
| Clean with betadine soaked gauze | | | | | |
| Dry with clean gauze | | | | | |

Practical

## Administer Local Anaesthetic

| | | | | | |
|---|---|---|---|---|---|
| Check date and dose of LA with a second person | | | | | |
| Draw up 5mls using a 21 gauge needle | | | | | |
| Dispose of needle in sharps | | | | | |
| Administer LA with a 25 gauge needle | | | | | |
| Ensures pulls back before administration to prevent intravenous administration | | | | | |
| Say would wait 5-10 minutes for LA to take affect | | | | | |

## Suturing

| | | | | | |
|---|---|---|---|---|---|
| Correctly hold needle holders and forceps | | | | | |
| Insert needle perpendicular to the skin at 5mm from wound edge, and exit at the middle of the wound | | | | | |
| Re-insert needle in middle of wound exiting 5mm from opposite edge to first insertion point | | | | | |
| Tie three surgical knots | | | | | |
| Position knot to one side of the wound, so it is not overlying the wound | | | | | |
| Repeat 5-10mm down the wound, alternating the position of the knot so that it is on the opposite side of the wound to the first knot | | | | | |
| Add as many sutures as required and ensure the wound edges are brought together | | | | | |

## Wound Aftercare

| | | | | | |
|---|---|---|---|---|---|
| Apply dressing | | | | | |
| Mention tetanus vaccine if not current or wound contaminated | | | | | |
| Advise patient to keep wound dry | | | | | |
| Education of signs of infection | | | | | |

Practical

---

**How long are sutures for simple lacerations kept in (excluding the face)?**

- 7 – 14 days

---

**What types of suture material are you aware of and give an example of each?**

- Absorbable and non-absorbable and each may be single filament or braided
- Absorbable monofilament = monocryl, PDS (polydioxanone)
- Absorbable braided = vicryl (polyglactin 910)
- Non-absorbable monofilament = prolene
- Non-absorbable braided = silk

---

**How long would you leave a suture on the face before removing?**

- Approximately 5 days

## What are the Royal College of Surgeons guidelines for achieving good anastomotic results for sutures?

- Tension free, opposing ends with no rotation, and a good blood supply (i.e. healthy tissue under no tension or stress)

## Additional Questions to Consider

1 // What is meant by aseptic technique?

2 // What additional issues might there be when suturing a child?

3 // When would you consider using glue to fix a head injury rather than sutures?

4 // What advice would you give the patient in terms of wound care after suturing it?

5 // What is a fasciotomy, and when would you use it?

Practical

# Chapter 6

# Radiology

*Candidate Briefing:* **Mr Taylor is 59 year man who has been sent in to hospital by his GP with worsening breathlessness and orthopnoea. Please describe the findings on the chest x-ray provided.**

CHEST X RAY 1 (taken from Unofficial Guide to Passing OSCEs 3rd Edition:, Chapter 6, Station 1)

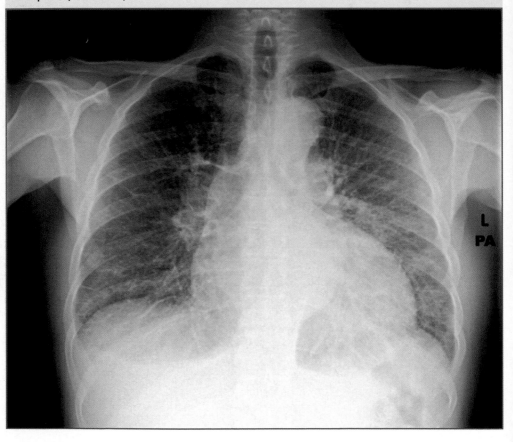

Additional Images to practice with:

*Candidate Briefing:* **A 75 year old man with progressive shortness of breath. Please present the findings of the chest X-ray and discuss further relevant investigations.**

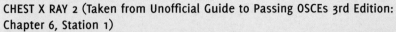

CHEST X RAY 2 (Taken from Unofficial Guide to Passing OSCEs 3rd Edition: Chapter 6, Station 1)

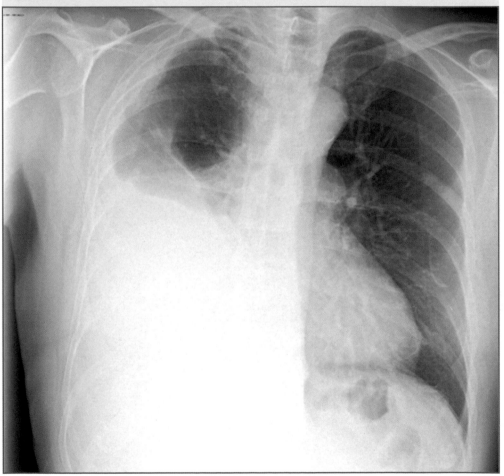

CHEST X RAY 3 (Taken from Unofficial Guide to Passing OSCEs 3rd Edition: Chapter 6, Station 1)

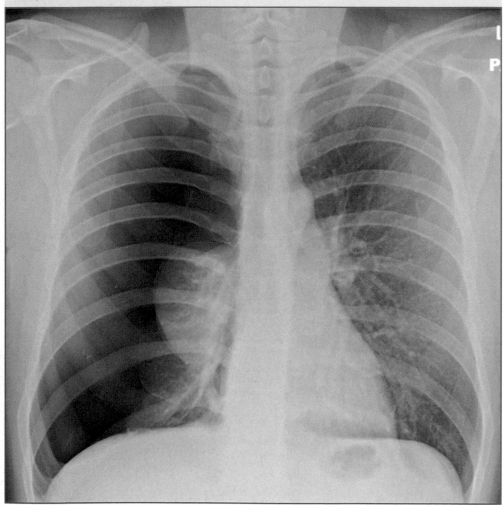

Radiology

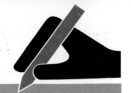

## Mark Scheme for Examiner

### Technical Aspects

| | | | | | |
|---|---|---|---|---|---|
| Checks patient details (name, date of birth, hospital number) | | | | | |
| Checks the date of the X-ray | | | | | |
| Identifies the projection of the X-ray | | | | | |
| Assesses technical quality of X-ray | | | | | |

### Obvious Abnormalities

| | | | | | |
|---|---|---|---|---|---|
| Describes any obvious abnormality | | | | | |
| Site (lung and zone/lobe) | | | | | |
| Size (if relevant) | | | | | |
| Shape (if relevant) | | | | | |
| Density | | | | | |

### Systematic Review of the Film

| | | | | | |
|---|---|---|---|---|---|
| Position of trachea | | | | | |
| Assessment of lungs | | | | | |
| Size and appearance of hila | | | | | |
| Assess for cardiomegaly (or states if this is not possible due to AP projection) | | | | | |
| Assesses cardiac borders and cardiophrenic angles | | | | | |
| Position and appearance of hemidiaphragms | | | | | |
| Evidence of pneumoperitoneum (free air under the diaphragm) | | | | | |
| Assesses the imaged skeleton | | | | | |
| Assesses the imaged soft tissues (e.g. surgical emphysema, mastectomy) | | | | | |
| Comments on iatrogenic abnormalities | | | | | |

Radiology

| Presents findings | | | | | |
|---|---|---|---|---|---|
| Reviews relevant previous imaging if appropriate | | | | | |
| Provides a differential diagnosis where appropriate | | | | | |
| Suggests appropriate further imaging/investigations if relevant | | | | | |

---

*Findings of Chest X Ray 1:*

This is a **PA** chest radiograph. **There are no identifying markings. I would like to ensure that it is the correct patient and to check the date that it was taken. It is a technically adequate film: it is not rotated, has adequate penetration, and good inspiratory effort. There are no important areas cut off at the edges of the film.**

There is marked cardiomegaly (cardiothoracic thoracic ratio 0.58) with upper lobe venous diversion. Kerley B lines are present. There are no pleural effusions.

Reviewing the rest of the film, the trachea is not deviated. Comparing the left and right lungs, I can see no other obvious abnormalities in the lung fields, such as consolidation. The hila are not enlarged. There is no evidence of pneumothaces. There is unfolding of the thoracic aorta causing widening of the left side of the mediastinum and a retrocardiac opacity. The heart borders are clear, as are the cardiophrenic angles. The diaphragms look normal, the costophrenic angles are clear, and there is no air under the diaphragm. The bones and imaged soft tissues are unremarkable, and there are no foreign bodies visable.

**In summary, this chest radiograph shows features of left ventricular failure. I would like to review previous chest x-rays if available to assess whether these findings have deteriorated. In addition he will need follow up chest x-rays after appropriate treatment has been commenced.**

## Findings of Chest X-ray 2:

This is an anonymised PA chest radiograph. The timing of the examination is also unavailable. The patient is slightly rotated to the left and X-ray is underpenetrated. It is still a diagnostic quality X-ray.

The most obvious abnormality is within the right hemithorax where there is homogenous increased opacification projected over the mid and lower zones of the right lung. The superior edge of the opacification is clearly defined and there is a meniscus evident. The right hemidiaphragm and cardiac border are obscured. There is minor linear atelectasis within the right upper zone.

Reviewing the rest of the film, the trachea is not deviated (allowing for the patient rotation). The left cardiac and mediastinal contours are normal. The left lung, left hilum and costophrenic angle are normal. No abnormality of the bony thorax or imaged soft tissues. No pneumoperitoneum.

**In summary, this chest X-ray shows a large right pleural effusion with associated atelectasis in the right upper zone. There is no other significant abnormality. Comparison with previous relevant imaging to assess the progression of the effusion would be helpful. Diagnostic aspiration should be considered +/- drainage if clinically appropriate. A repeat chest X-ray should be performed following these procedures to assess the size of the remaining effusion and presence of a pneumothorax.**

## Findings of Chest X-ray 3:

This is a PA chest radiograph. The patient details and timing of the examination have been removed. It is a technically adequate film: it is well centred, non-rotated, has adequate penetration and well inspired.

The most obvious abnormality is the large hyperlucent area within the right hemithorax. The edge of the right lung is clearly visible medial to this, with increased opacification of the visible right lung.

On review of the rest of the film, the trachea is central and there is no mediastinal shift or flattening of the hemidiaphragms. The left lung and hila are normal. The heart is not enlarged and the cardiac and mediastinal contours are normal. There is no blunting of the costophrenic angles to suggest pleural effusions. No free subdiaphragmatic gas. No fracture or subcutaneous emphysema.

**In summary, this chest X-ray shows a large right sided pneumothorax (>50%) with compressive atelectasis of the underlying right lung. There is no evidence of tension (no mediastinal shift or tracheal deviation). No cause for the pneumothorax is demonstrated on the X-ray. No previous relevant imaging is available for comparison. Repeat chest X-ray following appropriate intervention (chest drain insertion) is suggested.**

---

**What landmark would you use for inserting a chest drain in a large pleural effusion?**

- 5th intercostal space
- Mid-axillary line

---

**What is the upper limit of normal of the cardiothoracic ratio on a PA chest x-ray?**

- 0.5

---

**List 3 causes of pneumothorax?**

- Trauma
- Iatrogenic (e.g. post aspiration or percutaneous biopsy)
- Spontaneous
- Underlying lung disease (e.g. pulmonary fibrosis, cystic fibrosis, emphysema, PCP pneumonia)

1 // You are shown an X-ray with a large left sided pneumothorax. How would you manage this?

2 // Give three causes of a coin shaped lesion on a chest X-ray.

3 // How do you assess whether an chest X-ray is over or under penetrated?

4 // Name three causes of bronchiestasis.

5 // What tests might you order on a pleural tap to differentiate an exudate from a transudate? If you suspect malignancy what further tests on the pleural fluid might be helpful?

Radiology

*Candidate Briefing:* **Mr Pai is a 68-year-old gentleman who has presented with vomiting, abdominal pain, and a distended abdomen. He has not opened his bowels in one week, and has previously had bowel surgery. Describe the findings of the abdominal X-ray that is shown.**

ABDO X-RAY 1 (Taken from Unofficial Guide to Passing OSCEs 3rd Edition: Chapter 6, Station 2)

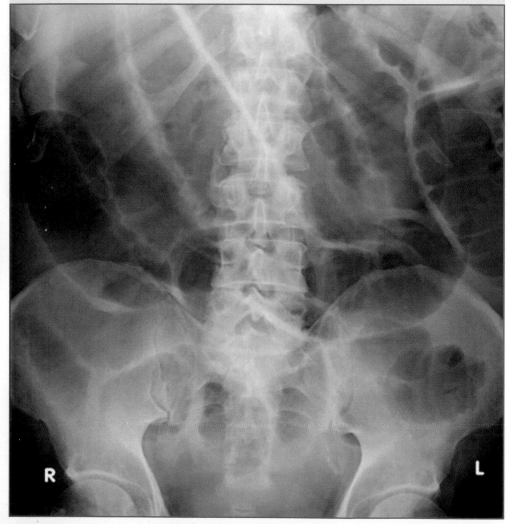

R

L

The Unofficial Guide to Passing OSCEs: *Candidate Briefings, Patient Briefings and Mark Schemes*

Additional Images to practice with:

*Candidate Briefing:* **Mrs Smith is an 83 year old woman who has presented with back pain. Please review and present the following X-ray. What further imaging would you consider?**

ABDO X-RAY 2 (Taken from Unofficial Guide to Passing OSCEs 3rd Edition: Chapter 6, Station 2)

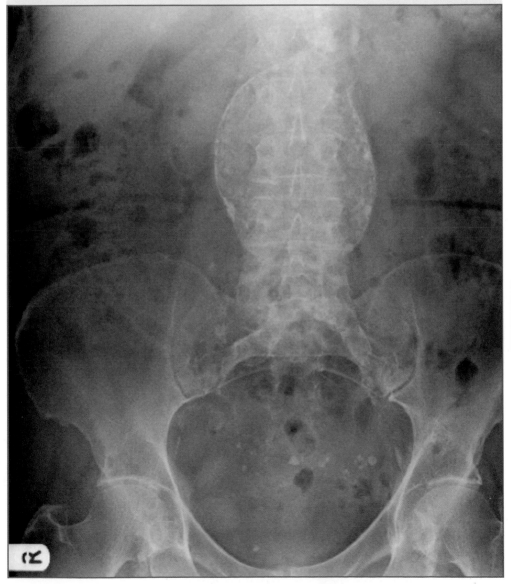

ABDO X-RAY 3 (Taken from Unofficial Guide to Passing OSCEs 3rd Edition: Chapter 6, Station 2)

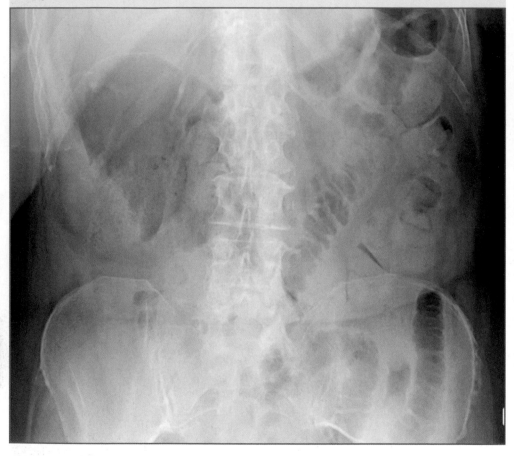

Radiology

# Mark Scheme for Examiner

## Technical Aspects

| | | | | | |
|---|---|---|---|---|---|
| Checks patient details (name, date of birth, hospital number) | | | | | |
| Checks the date of the X-ray | | | | | |
| Identifies the projection of the X-ray | | | | | |
| Assesses technical quality of X-ray | | | | | |

## Obvious Abnormalities

| | | | | | |
|---|---|---|---|---|---|
| Describes any obvious abnormality (site (e.g. large bowel), size, shape, density) | | | | | |

## Systematic Review of the Film

| | | | | | |
|---|---|---|---|---|---|
| Assesses the large bowel (diameter, wall thickening) | | | | | |
| Assesses small bowel (diameter, wall thickening) | | | | | |
| Comments of evidence of extraluminal gas (pneumoperitoneum) | | | | | |
| Comments on any abnormality of the liver, gallbladder or spleen (e.g. radio-opaque gallstones) | | | | | |
| Comments on any abnormality of the major vascular structures (aorta and iliac vessels) e.g. vascular calcification, aneurysm | | | | | |
| Assesses the urinary tract (kidney, ureters and bladder) e.g. calculi | | | | | |
| Assesses the imaged skeleton | | | | | |
| Comments on iatrogenic abnormalities (surgical clips, stents etc) | | | | | |

Radiology

## Summary

| | | | | | |
|---|---|---|---|---|---|
| Presents findings | | | | | |
| Reviews relevant previous imaging if appropriate | | | | | |
| Provides a differential diagnosis where appropriate | | | | | |
| Suggests appropriate further imaging/investigations if relevant | | | | | |

*Findings of Abdominal X-Ray 1:*

**This is an AP supine abdominal radiograph. There are no identifying markings. I would like to ensure that it is the correct patient and check the date it was taken. The upper abdomen and the lateral extremes of the patient are not included in this film.**

There are multiple dilated loops of small bowel. It is small bowel due to its predominantly central distribution and the presence of valvulae conniventes. There is no evidence of hernia or extraluminal gas. The abdominal aorta is not visible and the bladder appears normal in size. There are no apparent bony abnormalities.

**In summary, this is an abdominal radiograph showing small bowel obstruction with no evidence of perforation. I would like to arrange an erect CXR specifically to look for free air under the diaphragm. Differential diagnosis of the cause of small bowel obstruction includes adhesions, neoplasia, incarcerated hernia and strictures. Contrast enhanced CT of the abdomen and pelvis would allow further assessment of the site and cause of the small bowel obstruction.**

## Findings of Abdominal X-Ray 2:

This is a supine AP radiograph of the abdomen. It has been anonymised and the timing of the examination is not available. The left side of the abdomen has not been fully imaged.

Projected over the lumbar spine is a partially calcified structure which measures 4.3 cm in lateral diameter. Given its position and appearance it is most in keeping with a partially calcified abdominal aortic aneurysm. The outline of both psoas muscles is visible, suggesting there is no large retroperitoneal collection / haematoma.

The bowel gas pattern is normal. No plain film evidence of bowel obstruction, perforation or mucosal oedema. There are multiple rounded densities projected over the pelvis in keeping with calcified phleboliths. No significant abnormality of the imaged skeleton.

In summary this abdominal X-ray shows a partially calcified abdominal aortic aneurysm. I would like to review previous imaging to determine whether this is a new finding. Further appropriate imaging would depend on the clinical situation. An ultrasound could allow accurate measurement of the size of the aneurysm, however if there are clinical concerns over leaking or rupture of the aneurysm then a CT of the abdomen (pre-contrast and arterial phases) would be appropriate.

## Findings of Abdominal X-Ray 3:

This is a supine AP abdominal X-ray. The patient's details and timing of the examination have been removed. The entire pelvis and upper abdomen are not included on the X-ray.

Within the left lower quadrant there is a non-dilated loop of bowel. Both sides of the wall of this loop of bowel are clearly visible. This is in keeping with Rigler's sign (pneumoperitoneum).

The bowel gas pattern is normal with no plain film evidence of obstruction or mucosal oedema. No other significant abnormality evident within the imaged abdomen. No skeletal abnormality.

In summary this abdominal X-ray shows the presence of extraluminal gas. I would like to review the erect chest X-ray to confirm the presence of a pneumoperitoneum. The differential diagnosis of pneumoperitoneum is large but can be categorised as perforated viscus, iatrogenic (post operative) or rarely infective. The clinical condition will determine whether additional imaging is needed. Should it be required a CT of the abdomen and pelvis with IV contrast would be appropriate.

Radiology

---

### How would you manage small bowel obstruction?

- NBM
- IV fluids and NG tube
- Bloods (FBC, U/Es, CRP, clotting, group and save)
- Erect CXR
- Urgent surgical review regarding need for further imaging or surgery

---

### Name 3 causes of small bowel obstruction.

- Adhesions
- Hernias
- Tumours
- Volvulus
- Intussusception
- Foreign bodies
- Ischaemic strictures
- Gallstone ileus

---

### What is the maximum normal diameter of the small and large bowel on abdominal X-ray?

- Small bowel up to 3cm
- Large bowel up to 5cm (caecum can be up to 8cm)

Radiology

## List 4 causes of extraluminal gas within the abdominal cavity.

- Perforated viscus (ulcer, diverticulum, tumour, ischaemia, inflammatory bowel disease)
- Post operative
- Penetrating trauma
- Gas forming infections
- Gas from chest (eg bronchopleural fistula) or vagina

## Additional Questions to Consider

1 // Define the term 'aneurysm' and discuss the management options of an abdominal aortic aneurysm.

2 // How do you differentiate between large and small bowel obstruction on an X-ray?

3 // Discuss how you would manage a sigmoid volvulus causing obstruction.

4 // Discuss the causes of bowel wall/mucosal oedema. Which potentially lethal large bowel complication of mucosal oedema is often screened for using abdominal X-rays?

5 // Name three causes of large bowel obstruction.

Radiology

*Candidate Briefing:* **Mrs Jones is a 68-year-old lady who has recently fallen. Her leg is shortened and externally rotated. Tell the radiologist what films you would like to request, and then describe the findings of the film that is shown.**

ORTHOPAEDIC X-RAY 1: (Taken from Unofficial Guide to Passing OSCEs 3rd Edition: Chapter 6, Station 3)

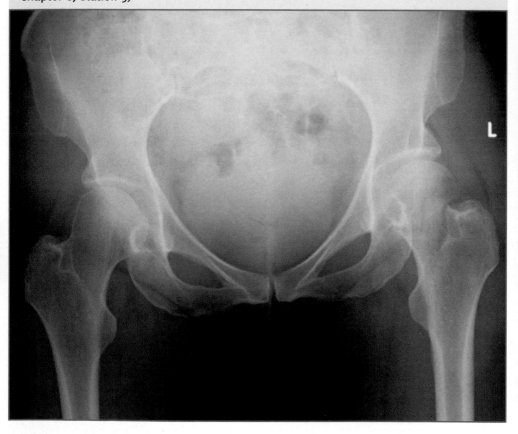

Radiology

Additional Images to practice with:

*Candidate Briefing:* **Miss Walker caught her little finger in a door and has presented with an obvious deformity. Please describe the X-ray findings. Are there any other views you would like to review?**

ORTHOPAEDIC X-RAY 2: (Taken from Unofficial Guide to Passing OSCEs 3rd Edition: Chapter 6, Station 3)

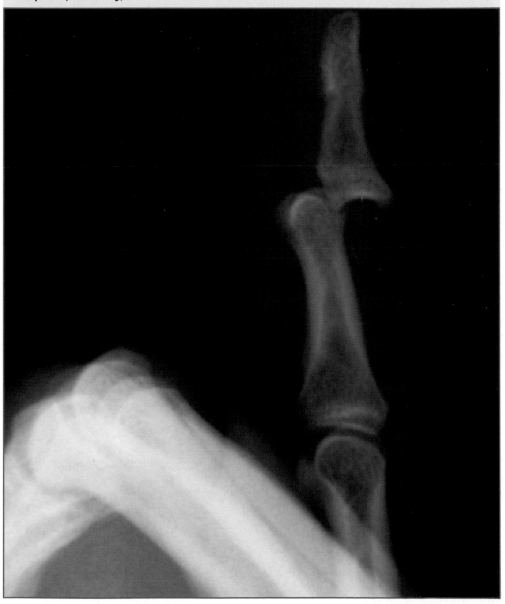

ORTHOPAEDIC X-RAY 3: (Taken from Unofficial Guide to Passing OSCEs 3rd Edition: Chapter 6, Station 3)

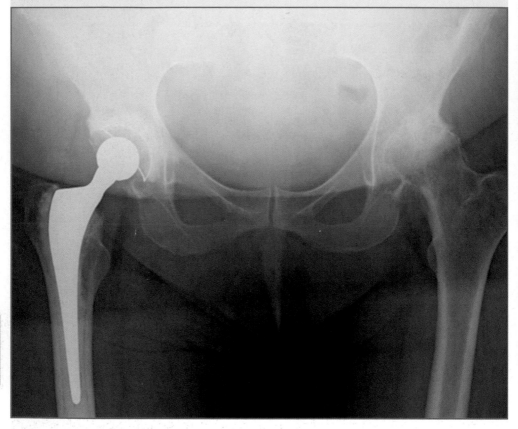

Radiology

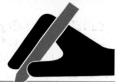

# Mark Scheme for Examiner

## Technical Aspects

| | | | | | |
|---|---|---|---|---|---|
| Checks patient details (name, date of birth, hospital number) | | | | | |
| Checks the date of the X-ray | | | | | |
| Identifies the projection of the X-ray | | | | | |
| Assesses technical quality of X-ray (entire bone/joint included, adequate views) | | | | | |

## Obvious Abnormalities

| | | | | | |
|---|---|---|---|---|---|
| Describes any obvious abnormality | | | | | |
| Systematic review of the film | | | | | |
| Assesses the bones for fractures (cortical step, buckle, gap, disruption of the trabeculae, disruption of Shenton's Line) | | | | | |
| Comments on the joints (dislocation / subluxation) | | | | | |
| Assesses for joint effusions if appropriate (e.g. knee or elbow) | | | | | |
| Comments on degenerative joint changes | | | | | |
| Comment on abnormal bone texture (e.g. radiolucency consistent with osteopenia) | | | | | |

## Describing fractures (if relevant)

| | | | | | |
|---|---|---|---|---|---|
| Which bone | | | | | |
| Which part of the bone (proximal, middle, distal third, intra-articular) | | | | | |
| Fracture pattern (simple / open, comminuted, impacted) | | | | | |
| Fracture type (transverse, oblique, spiral, greenstick) | | | | | |
| Displacement | | | | | |
| Angulation | | | | | |

Radiology

| | | | | | |
|---|---|---|---|---|---|
| Rotation | | | | | |
| Shortening | | | | | |

## Summary

| | | | | | |
|---|---|---|---|---|---|
| Presents findings | | | | | |
| Reviews relevant previous imaging if appropriate | | | | | |
| Provides a differential diagnosis where appropriate | | | | | |
| Suggests appropriate further imaging / investigations if relevant | | | | | |

---

*Findings of Orthopaedic X-Ray 1:*

**This is an AP Pelvis radiograph. There are no identifying markings. I would like to ensure that this is the correct patient and check the date that it was taken. The film is not rotated and there are no important areas cut off at the edges of the film.**

There is an oblique intracapsular fracture involving the left femoral neck. It is a simple fracture with minimal displacement. There is no angulation, rotation or shortening. There is no intra-articular involvement. Bone lucency is normal.

**There are no other abnormalities on the radiograph. A lateral X-ray is needed to complete the radiological assessment of the fracture.**

---

*Findings of Orthopaedic X-Ray 2:*

**This is a lateral view of the 5th finger. The patient details and timing of the examination are not available. The proximal aspect of the digit is obscured by the other fingers.**

There is posterior dislocation of the distal phalanx of the 5th digit. No fracture is visible on this single view. To complete my assessment I would like to review an AP view of the digit.

**Repeat AP and lateral views should be performed following manipulation of the digit.**

*Findings of Orthopaedic X-Ray 3:*

This is an anonymised AP X-ray of the pelvis. It is a technically adequate X-ray of the hips.

There is marked degenerative change at the left hip joint, with complete loss of joint space, subchondral sclerosis, osetophytes and bone cysts. No fracture is visible.

There is a right total hip replacement. No periprosthetic fracture is visible. No obvious loosening of the prosthesis, although I would like to compare with previous films to thoroughly assess the position of the prosthesis.

In summary this single AP view of the pelvis shows marked degenerative changes at the left hip joint and a right total hip replacement. No fracture is visible. I would like to review a lateral film of the symptomatic hip, as well as previous pelvic X-rays to complete my assessment.

## Questions And Answers for Candidate

### What four signs on an X-ray might suggest osteoarthritis?

- Reduced joint space
- Osteophyte formation
- Subchondral sclerosis
- Subchondral cyst formation

### What does a fat fluid level on a horizontal beam lateral knee X-ray signify?

- Lipohaemarthrosis from a possible intracapsular fracture

Radiology

In the context of trauma, which views are required for a technically adequate X-ray assessment of the cervical spine?

- Lateral view showing C1 to the C7/T1 disc space
- AP view
- Open mouth PEG view showing C1/C2 articulation

## Additional Questions to Consider

1 // What further views / imaging could be used to assess the cervical spine if the standard 3-view assessment is inadequate?

2 // What is the difference between subluxation and dislocation?

3 // Discuss the blood supply to the femoral head and its relevance to the treatment of neck of femur fractures.

4 // How would you manage an open fracture of the midshaft of the radius?

5 // Which bones are particularly at risk of avascular necrosis following a fracture?

# Chapter 7

# Obstetrics And Gynaecology

# Station 1
## PLACENTA PRAEVIA

*Candidate Briefing:* **Ms Jones is a 26 year-old lady who is 20 weeks pregnant in her first pregnancy. Her routine abnormality ultrasound scan demonstrates placenta praevia. Her husband works overseas and she has come to clinic to discuss the result of her scan. Please explain the scan result to her, including a discussion of the risks associated with this condition and how this may be managed.**

*Patient Briefing:* **You are Ms Jones. You are 26 years old and 20 weeks pregnant in your first pregnancy. You have just had your 20 week scan and have been told there is something wrong with the placenta, you can't remember what it is called, but you are aware that you are in clinic to discuss this. You have had no bleeding in the pregnancy so far.**

If asked you are concerned about whether this carries any risk to the pregnancy. During the consultation you will be given information from the doctor. If they say anything which you don't understand or they use medical language look at them confused. Do not interrupt them to say you don't understand but if they specifically offer you the opportunity to ask questions or ask if you understand you should then ask them to go over those areas.

**If they ask your rhesus status or blood group, answer you are 'A Negative'. If asked you are living with your sister because your husband is temporarily working overseas.**

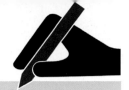

## Introduction

Clean hands, introduce self, confirm patient identity

Check identity of others in the room and confirm that the patient is happy for them to be present

Establish current patient knowledge and concerns

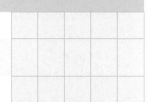

## Translation of Information

Explains placenta praevia in simple terms (using diagrams if necessary)

## Bleeding

Explains may not have any symptoms at all

Explains about the increased risk of bleeding

Advise admission to hospital in the event of a bleed

Explain that bleeding may be heavy which could endanger patient and baby, and may require emergency treatment (including a C Section)

Explain that recurrent bleeding in later pregnancy may require long term admission to hospital until delivery

Ask about rhesus status, if rhesus negative explain that Anti D will need to be given if there is a bleed

Management of delivery

Explains that as the pregnancy progresses the placenta may move away from the opening of the womb

Offer to assess placental location by ultrasound at 36 weeks

Explain delivery options (vaginal delivery vs caesarean)

O&G

## Finishing the Consultation

| | | | | |
|---|---|---|---|---|
| Elicit patient concerns or questions | | | | |
| Ask about current living circumstances / support network | | | | |
| Summarise back to the patient | | | | |
| Arrange a follow up appointment (as necessary) or offer your contact details | | | | |
| Thank patient and close consultation | | | | |

## General Points

| | | | | |
|---|---|---|---|---|
| Check patient understands regularly, and offer information leaflets | | | | |
| Maintain good eye contact and engage with patient | | | | |
| Avoid medical jargon | | | | |
| Polite to patient | | | | |

## Questions And Answers for Candidate

### How would you differentiate a minor and a major placenta praevia? What is the significance in terms of delivery options?

- Minor: the placenta is in the lower segment, near to (or touching) the os, there is a potential for vaginal delivery (depending on the distance of the lower edge of placenta from the internal os)
- Major: the placenta is completely or partially covering the os, caesarean section is required (vaginal delivery not possible)

## What is the major risk with placenta praevia?

- The risk of placenta praevia is a sudden, major haemorrhage, which can threaten the life of both the mother and the fetus

## Why does placenta praevia seen on the 20 week anomaly scan resolve by 36 weeks in the majority of cases?

- The uterus grows upward from the cervix as the pregnancy progresses; this results in the formation of the lower segment of the uterus and effectively means that the placenta 'moves up' with advancing gestation

## State two risk factor for placenta praevia.

- Increasing maternal age and previous caesarean section, previous uterine surgery, IVF, smoking, twin pregnancy, previous placenta praevia

## Additional Questions to Consider

1 // What investigation is used to monitor placenta praevia?

2 // What is placenta accreta and state the three forms.

3 // Define vasa praevia.

4 // If the placenta praevia resulted in a large antepartum haemorrhage at 32 weeks gestation, how would you manage it?

5 // What would you advise the mother to abstain from if she has a diagnosis of placenta praevia?

O&G

# Station 2
## BREECH PRESENTATION

*Candidate Briefing:* **Mrs Rae is 37 weeks pregnant and has been diagnosed as having a frank breech presentation of her first pregnancy. Please explain the diagnosis. Then discuss the possibility of external cephalic version (ECV) to put the baby into a normal position, and delivery options if ECV is unsuccessful.**

*Patient Briefing:* **You are Mrs Rae. You are 37 weeks into your first pregnancy. You have just had a scan and you have been told your baby is facing the wrong way, and have now been asked to see the doctor to discuss this.**

If asked you are concerned because you don't know if there is something wrong with the baby, and you are anxious to find out what this means for your pregnancy. The questions below are for you to ask if the doctor does not cover them and they offer you the chance to ask questions:
*What is the safest way for me to deliver my baby?*
*If ECV carries risks, is it not safer to just have a caesarean section?*
*My friend gave birth to their child bottom first and they had no problems, can I just deliver bottom first?*

**Throughout the station the doctor will pass on information to you. If there are any areas which they explain in a confusing manner or use complex medical language, look confused. Do not interrupt the doctor but if they allow you time to ask questions ask them to clarify these areas for you.**

O&G

7 // Obstetrics And Gynaecology    The Unofficial Guide to Passing OSCEs: *Candidate Briefings, Patient Briefings and Mark Schemes*

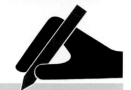

## Mark Scheme for Examiner

### Introduction

Clean hands, introduce self, confirm patient identity

Check identity of others in the room and confirm that the patient is happy for them to be present

Establish current patient knowledge and concerns

### Translation of Information

Explain breech presentation, including cause, simple terms

Explain potential problems with breech vaginal delivery

Explain ECV (external cephalic version) in simple terms and why it is done

Explain the risks associated with ECV

Explain what happens if ECV fails or if it is declined

### Finishing the Consultation

Elicit patient concerns or questions

Summarise back to the patient

Arrange a follow up appointment (as necessary) or offer your contact details

Thank patient and close consultation

### General Points

Check patient understands regularly, and offer information leaflets

Maintain good eye contact and engage with patient

Avoid medical jargon

Polite to patient

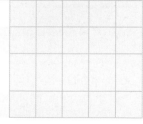

---

## How common is breech presentation at term?

- Between 2-5%

---

## State 2 conditions that increase the risk of breech presentation.

- Multiple pregnancy
- Fibroids
- Placenta praevia
- Fetal anomaly
- Polyhydramnios
- Oligohydramnios

---

## State 3 contraindications for ECV

- Abnormal CTG
- Major uterine anomaly
- Antepartum haemorrhage within the last 7 days
- Ruptured membranes
- Multiple pregnancy (except for delivery of twin 2) and where caesarean section is required regardless of presentation

321

7 // Obstetrics And Gynaecology    The Unofficial Guide to Passing OSCEs: *Candidate Briefings, Patient Briefings and Mark Schemes*

1 // Explain the difference between extended, flexed and footling breech presentation.

2 // What complication should you be particularly wary of in a footling presentation, compared to other presentations?

3 // When should ECV be offered?

4 // When might you consider a vaginal delivery for a breech presentation?

5 // For a paediatrician doing the baby check, of what orthopedic problem is a breech presentation baby at an increased risk?

*Candidate Briefing:* **Mrs Taylor is pregnant at term with her first child. Her foetus has a breech presentation. Delivery options have been discussed and she is considering an elective caesarean section. Please explain the risks and benefits of this procedure to her.**

*Patient Briefing:* **You are Mrs Taylor. You are pregnant at term with your first baby. You are aware that you have come to discuss the mode of delivery with the doctor. You are aware that your baby is breech and that this can make vaginal birth more difficult.**

If you are asked about your concerns you respond *'I just want the best for my baby'. I have been told I can try and deliver vaginally or I can have a caesarean but I don't know what to do'.* If the doctor says anything that to a lay person may sound gruesome when describing the caesarean section please jump back in your seat and look horrified. Unless they make it very clear ask them if it will hurt during the operation.

**If there are any areas during the conversation where the doctor fails to clearly explain a point or uses complex medical language you are to look confused. Do not interrupt the doctor but if they allow you time to ask questions get them to clarify the point for you.**

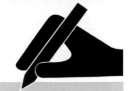

## Introduction

Clean hands, introduce self, confirm patient identity

Check identity of others in the room and confirm that the patient is happy for them to be present

Establish current patient knowledge and concerns

## Translation of Information

Explains indication for caesarean section

Explains in simple terms what a caesarean is and how it is done

Explain major risks of procedure: bleeding (1:5000 severe needing hysterectomy), infection (1:20), blood clot (1:1000), injury to organs (1:1000)

Additional risks: post-operative pain, ileus, 50% risk of another caesarean section in a future pregnancy

Risks to baby: breathing difficulty at birth, cuts to the babies skin

## Finishing the Consultation

Elicit patient concerns or questions

Summarise back to the patient

Arrange a follow up appointment (as necessary) or offer your contact details

Thank patient and close consultation

O&G

## General Points

| | | | | |
|---|---|---|---|---|
| Check patient understands regularly, and offer information leaflets | | | | |
| Maintain good eye contact and engage with patient | | | | |
| Avoid medical jargon | | | | |
| Polite to patient | | | | |

## Questions And Answers for Candidate

### How do we reduce the risk of blood clots after caesarean section (3 points)?

- Low molecular weight heparin
- TED stockings
- Encourage mobilisation

### List 3 reasons why caesarean section might be performed.

- Placenta praevia
- Severe IUGR
- Severe pre-eclampsia
- Breech presentation
- Placental abruption
- Maternal choice
- Previous caesarean section
- Mother unsuitable for a vaginal delivery etc (many different answers possible but these are the most common reasons)

## What is the most commonly performed incision for a caesarean section?

- Transverse incision lower (uterine) segment caesarean section

## Additional Questions to Consider

1 // What are the key aspects of preparing a patient for a caesarean section?

2 // Name the 3 forms of anaesthesia that might be considered for a woman undergoing a caesarean section.

3 // What drug is given intravenously to aid uterine contraction and why?

4 // What risk is there to the baby from a caesarean section?

5 // What is the rough incidence of DVT / PE developing post operatively?

O&G

# Station 4
# ANTEPARTUM HAEMORRHAGE

*Candidate Briefing:* **Mrs Patel is 30 weeks pregnant. She has noticed blood passing from her vagina and is very concerned. Please take a history from her and establish a differential diagnosis.**

*Patient Briefing:* **You are Mrs Patel. You are 30 weeks pregnant. You will act very anxious when the doctor enters the room. You have come to see the doctor because you have passed blood from down below (state vagina if doctor asks for clarification).**

If asked about your concerns you are very concerned about the health of the baby, and are worried you could be losing baby.

When asked to give more detail about what happened state "I started bleeding about 11:00am yesterday morning and the bleeding has been on and off for over 24 hours now. The blood is bright red. I am very scared." After this only answer direct questions.
In total you guess you have lost about a large coffee mug of blood. You are now wearing a pad to check blood loss and there has been none since you arrived here. There have not been any clots.

Today you have felt some fairly severe cramping lower abdominal pains that feel like severe period pains, but at the moment you are comfortable. You were lying in bed when the bleeding first started and there is nothing you can think of that has brought it on. You have not felt baby moving much since yesterday.

No previous pregnancies. If asked you believe you are rhesus positive.
No previous medical or surgical history, on no medication, no allergies, non smoker, no alcohol. You currently live alone as your husband has recently left you.

*When asked directly if there is anything else you would like to mention, say that you do not know if it's important but both your sisters have bled heavily during and after delivery of their children.*

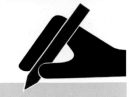

## Introduction

Clean hands, introduce self, confirm patient identity

Check identity of others in the room and confirm that the patient is happy for them to be present

Establish current patient knowledge and concerns

## Presenting Complaint

Assess amount of bleeding

Is the patient passing clots

Precipitating factors

Associated pain

Foetal movements

## Current Pregnancy

Scans – specifically identify placental location

Complications in this pregnancy

Rhesus status

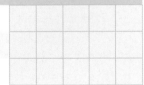

## History

Past obstetric history – number of pregnancies, method of delivery, outcome of pregnancies and any complications

Past medical, surgical and social history

Drug history and allergies

Asks if there is any other information the patient would like to offer

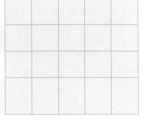

## Finishing the Consultation

| | | | | | |
|---|---|---|---|---|---|
| Elicit patient concerns or questions | | | | | |
| Summarise back to the patient | | | | | |
| Arrange a follow up appointment (as necessary) or offer your contact details | | | | | |
| Thank patient and close consultation | | | | | |

## General Points

| | | | | | |
|---|---|---|---|---|---|
| Check patient understands regularly, and offer information leaflets | | | | | |
| Maintain good eye contact and engage with patient | | | | | |
| Avoid medical jargon | | | | | |
| Polite to patient | | | | | |

## Questions And Answers for Candidate

### If this patient had presented to you bleeding very heavily, how would you begin managing her?

- Resuscitate using an ABCDE approach
- 2 large bore IV cannulas and IV fluids
- Bloods - FBC, clotting and crossmatch
- Once mother is stable assess fetal well-being – CTG/ Ultrasound scan
- Senior obstetric review

### What is the definition of an antepartum haemorrhage?

- Vaginal bleeding from 24 weeks gestation until the onset of labour

### Why might the amount of vaginal bleeding not reflect the true amount of bleeding in a placental abruption?

- Vaginal blood loss is the amount of revealed bleeding only, not the internal retroplacental bleeding (concealed bleeding)

## Additional Questions to Consider

1 // **What is the classical abdominal examination finding in the case of abruption?**

2 // **In the case of a major bleed with placental abruption what is the ultimate treatment?**

3 // **State one relatively common cause of local bleeding from the cervix.**

4 // **What important consideration should you take in rhesus negative women with antepartum hemorrhage?**

5 // **What are the most common causes of antepartum hemorrhage?**

O&G

# Station 5
## OBSTETRIC EXAMINATION

*Candidate Briefing:* **Mrs Pfannenstiel is 32 weeks pregnant. Please perform an obstetric examination and present your findings.**

*Patient Briefing:* **You are 32 weeks pregnant Mrs Pfannensteil. You are happy to be examined by the doctor and follow their instructions. If they do not tell you what they are doing at each stage through the examination ask them 'what are you doing?' If the doctor's examination technique is painful grimace and let out a quiet aghh. If the doctor apologises accept their apology.**

## Mark Scheme for Examiner

### Introduction

| | | | | | |
|---|---|---|---|---|---|
| Clean hands, introduce self, confirm patient identity, and gain consent | | | | | |
| Position patient comfortably at 45° | | | | | |

### Examination

| | | | | | |
|---|---|---|---|---|---|
| Obtains adequate exposure | | | | | |
| General inspection of patient, general appearance, oedema, look for pallor | | | | | |
| Measures symphysio-fundal height | | | | | |
| Assess fetal lie | | | | | |
| Assess fetal presentation | | | | | |
| Assess engagement | | | | | |
| Auscultate fetal heart rate | | | | | |

| | | | | | |
|---|---|---|---|---|---|
| Review observations | | | | | |
| Assess reflexes | | | | | |
| Feel for clonus | | | | | |
| Palpate calves | | | | | |
| Auscultate chest | | | | | |
| Feel for peripheral oedema | | | | | |
| Perform vaginal / speculum examination | | | | | |

## General

| | | | | | |
|---|---|---|---|---|---|
| Progressed speedily with confidence | | | | | |
| Communicates clear instructions to patient | | | | | |
| Minimises pain and makes patient feel at ease | | | | | |

## Questions And Answers for Candidate

### Name 3 possible presentations of the fetus

- Cephalic
- Brow
- Face
- Breech
- Limb

## Which is the most unstable lie?

- Oblique

## For what reasons might the fetal head not engage? Give two reasons.

- Pelvic inlet too small
- Fetal head too big (macrosomia, fetal head malformation)
- Breech presentation (or abnormal lie)
- Placenta praevia
- Uterine abnormality (fibroids, bicornate uterus)
- Multiparous pregnancy (may not engage until labour)

**?** Additional Questions to Consider

1 // When measuring symphysio-fundal height, how much would you expect the uterus to grow each week of gestation?

2 // Why might the symphysio-fundal height measurement be inconsistent with gestational age? Give two reasons.

3 // Why is obesity problematic in an obstetric examination?

4 // What clinical signs might you find in pre-eclampsia?

# Station 6
# ANXIOUS PREGNANT WOMAN

*Candidate Briefing:* **Mrs Brown is a 44 year-old primigravida who has presented to your GP practice after having had a positive home pregnancy test. She is very anxious about her pregnancy. Please explore her anxieties and establish whether her pregnancy is high or low risk.**

---

*Patient Briefing:* **You are Mrs Brown, a 44 year old lady who has yesterday taken a positive pregnancy test after missing her period. This is your second pregnancy (previous miscarriage at 10 weeks). You will appear extremely anxious to the doctor, initially fidgeting on your chair and not making eye contact. You will also only answer with very short answers to questions initially.**

If the doctor attempts to console you and give reassurance you will relax, make good eye contact and hold a better conversation. When asked why you have attended today you explain that your period was 2 weeks late so you did a pregnancy test yesterday which was positive.

If asked about your current ideas about what happens next you reply 'I have no idea, I just don't know what to do.'

When asked specifically about possible concerns explain that you 'want to keep the pregnancy, but you haven't told your husband about it yet and you are scared that he will not want to keep it.' If questioned further explain that you tried IVF nearly 10 years ago but without success so you and your husband had abandoned the idea of children.' If the doctor makes an attempt at reassurance here again relax further and be fully co-operative for the rest of the consultation.

No surgical history, no medications, no allergies. Non-smoker, no alcohol, no housing or social concerns. You live with your husband and have close friends who live nearby.

*When asked about details of your pregnancy and medical history:*
*LMP – 6 weeks ago*
*Unplanned pregnancy, not taken any folic acid*
*No complications of pregnancy so far*
*Medical history of aortic regurgitation and type 1 diabetes mellitus. Your mother told you there is also a strong family history of congenital heart diseases but you don't know any other information about it.*

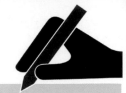

## Mark Scheme for Examiner

### Introduction

| Clean hands, introduce self, confirm patient identity | | | | |
|---|---|---|---|---|
| Check identity of others in the room and confirm that the patient is happy for them to be present | | | | |

### Ideas, Concerns, Expectations

| Ideas: establish why the patient has attended; enquires about what they already know about the process | | | | |
|---|---|---|---|---|
| Concerns: establish patient concerns | | | | |
| Asks about other potential concerns not volunteered e.g. Does the patient wish to continue the pregnancy? Early pregnancy symptoms. Social / housing concerns | | | | |
| Expectations: establishes patients current awareness of next steps for her pregnancy / help available | | | | |

### Assess Pregnancy Risk

| Current pregnancy: age, LMP, folic acid, planned / unplanned | | | | |
|---|---|---|---|---|
| Problems in pregnancy so far | | | | |
| Past obstetric history – gravida, parity, pregnancy outcomes and complication | | | | |
| Past medical and surgical history | | | | |
| Drug history and allergy status | | | | |
| Social history: alcohol, smoking, social support | | | | |
| Asks if there is any other information the patient would like to offer | | | | |

Summarise back to the patient, explain 'risk of pregnancy' and support provided for the pregnancy by health care professionals

Arrange a follow up appointment (as necessary) or offer your contact details

Thank patient and close consultation

## General Points

Check patient understands regularly, and offer information leaflets

Maintain good eye contact and engage with patient

Avoid medical jargon

Polite to patient

## Questions And Answers for Candidate

### If the patient were of Afro-Carribean origin, what haemoglobinopathies might you consider?

- Sickle cell
- Thalassemia

> **What is the risk of miscarriage if a woman undergoes amnio-centesis or chorionic villous sampling?**

- 1% for amniocentesis and 2% if undergoing chorionic villous sampling

> **When screening for Down syndrome with an ultrasound scan, what is the clinician looking for?**

- Nuchal translucency

## Additional Questions to Consider

1 // Why is folic acid important before conception and during pregnancy?

2 // If this lady is pregnant and chooses to go ahead with the pregnancy when should she ideally have her booking visit?

3 // What is the purpose of the antenatal booking visit?

4 // List 3 common causes of infertility.

5 // If this lady was pregnant and wanted to go ahead with an abortion at this stage, describe the medical and surgical management options.

*Candidate Briefing:* **Miss Williams is a 36 year-old lady in a long-term relationship. She is looking to start using the combined oral contraceptive pill as her partner no longer wishes to use condoms – she worries about the risk of future pregnancy. Please counsel her as to what this would mean for her and establish whether she is suitable for this form of contraception.**

*Patient Briefing:* **You are Miss Williams. You are 36 years old. You are in a stable long term relationship and have attended to enquire about the combined contraceptive pill.**

You have looked on the internet about various methods of contraception and you think the combined pill is right for you but would like some more information about it. The reason you are looking to change contraception is that you are now in a stable relationship and both yourself and your partner would like to stop using condoms to achieve a heightened sexual experience. You want a contraception method that is easy to stop if the side effects become too much. You have friends who have had bad experiences with the Mirena coil and depot injections so you refuse to consider these options. If asked about vasectomy explain that your husband said 'he refuses to let anyone go near his genitals with anything sharp'.

When asked about medical history:
Cycles – regular every 28 days, bleed heavily for 6 days but periods are not painful.
2 normal vaginal deliveries from a previous relationship. No STIs, normal smear history. You have only ever used condoms or abstinence for contraception. No past medical, surgical, drug or family history of note. No allergies. Social history – non smoker, occasional alcohol (6 units a week on further questioning), normal BMI.

*Questions you can ask if not explained by the doctor: When is it best to start taking the pill? How reliable is the pill? What do I do if I miss a pill?*

## Mark Scheme for Examiner

## Introduction

Clean hands, introduce self, confirm patient identity

Check identity of others in the room and confirm that the patient is happy for them to be present

Establish current patient knowledge and concerns

Briefly discusses modes of contraception available

## Establishes Patient Suitability for the Pill

Gynaecology history: menstrual cycle – length, regularity, pain and bleeding, contraceptive history, sexual health history, smear history

Medical and surgical history

Drug history and allergy status

Family history – breast Ca and venous thrombosis

Social history – specifically smoking and BMI

## Translation of Information

Explain briefly how the pill works

How to take the pill (daily for 21 days, 7 day break); when to start taking the pill (1st-5th day of cycle, or start anytime and use condoms for 7 days)

Benefit of the pill (effectiveness, ease of use, lightening periods, reduced cancer risks)

Major side effects: blood clots, migraines, high blood pressure

Minor side effects: weight gain, dizziness, nausea, breast tenderness, mood swings

Missed pill: what to do if one pill or two pills missed

States to be aware of medicine interactions

Advise that pill doesn't protect against STIs (and discusses other methods)

## Finishing the Consultation

Elicit patient concerns or questions

Summarise back to the patient

Arrange a follow up appointment (as necessary) or offer your contact details

Thank patient and close consultation

## General Points

Check patient understands regularly, and offer information leaflets

Maintain good eye contact and engage with patient

Avoid medical jargon

Polite to patient

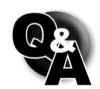

## Questions And Answers for Candidate

### What advice would you give the patient if she develops vomiting or diarrhoea?

- Your body may not have absorbed the pill, use alternative contraception for the duration of the illness and 7 days after

## What is the mechanism for the COC pill?

- Inhibits ovulation, makes the endometrium less favourable to support a fertilized egg, and makes the cervical mucus thicker

## Name 1 form of cancer which the COC pill reduces the risk of.

- Ovarian or endometrial cancer

## ? Additional Questions to Consider

1 // Name 3 drugs which interact with the COC pill.

2 // If a woman is already on the pill tell me three things you must check in a follow-up visit.

3 // State three other forms of contraception that could be used by a woman.

4 // How do you manage a woman who was taking the COC pill and suffers a DVT?

5 // Discuss why for social reasons the COC pill may not be suitable for some women.

*Candidate Briefing:* **Sarah is a 16 year-old female who had unprotected intercourse last night, and is worried she may be pregnant. Please advise her as to what her options are with regard to emergency contraception and explain the risks and benefits of different methods.**

*Patient Briefing:* **You are Sarah, a timid 16 year old who is worried she may be pregnant. You explain when asked that you have come to the doctors to have emergency treatment because there is a chance you have fallen pregnant because you had unprotected intercourse last night.**

If asked this occurred because you and your boyfriend were horny and you had run out of condoms. If asked what you know already you explain that there is a pill you can take which if taken early can prevent pregnancy.

Further history: Intercourse was at 10 pm last night. LMP 3 weeks ago, usually regular 28 day cycles. Contraception history: condoms only, occasionally you forget to use them. Previous chlamydia infection 6 months ago which was treated at the GUM clinic. 1 regular 17 year old partner for 1 year. No past medical surgical or drug history. No allergies.

**Questions to ask if not covered by doctor: Is there any other treatment available other than the pill? Will this cover me against catching infections as well?**

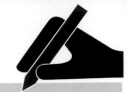

## Mark Scheme for Examiner

### Introduction

Clean hands, introduce self, confirm patient identity

Check identity of others in the room and confirm that the patient is happy for them to be present

Establish current patient knowledge and concerns

### Brief History

When was the unprotected intercourse

Gynaecological history – LMP, contraception, previous STIs

Past medical history, pregnancies, medications, allergies, social history

### Translation of Information

Briefly describe the 2 options available, explain if one is contra-indicated from information gathered from history

Explain levonelle: how it works, success rate, when to take second dose (if vomits in three hours), and side effects; need to take pregnancy test if no period for 3 weeks

Explain IUD: when it can be used, effectiveness, when it is removed. Risks at insertion, and risks whilst implanted

Follow up: neither method protects against STIs, advise GUM clinic 2 weeks after intercourse

### Finishing the Consultation

Elicit patient concerns or questions

Summarise back to the patient

Arrange a follow up appointment (as necessary) or offer your contact details

Thank patient and close consultation

| Check patient understands regularly, and offer information leaflets | | | | | |
|---|---|---|---|---|---|
| Maintain good eye contact and engage with patient | | | | | |
| Avoid medical jargon | | | | | |
| Polite to patient | | | | | |

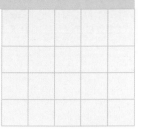

### If the patient was under 16, could the patient give consent to treatment?

Yes. For contraception they must meet the following criteria (Fraser guidelines):
• Will understand the advice
• Cannot be persuaded to inform parents / allow you to inform parents
• Is very likely to continue having sexual intercourse with or without contraceptive treatment
• That unless she receives contraceptive advice or treatment her physical or mental health or both are likely to suffer
• That her best interests require contraceptive advice, treatment or both without the parental consent

### Name two methods of emergency contraception currently available.

• Progesterone pill (levonelle)
• Ulipristal
• Copper IUD

O&G

> **What is the longest period after unprotected sexual intercourse that progesterone-only emergency contraception can be effectively given?**

- 3 days for levonelle (ulipristal can be given up to 5 days)

 **Additional Questions to Consider**

1 // State 3 of the symptoms and signs for chlamydia.

2 // How is chlamydia treated?

3 // What differential diagnoses would you give for a woman with increased amount of vaginal discharge that smells different?

4 // What are some difficulties perceived by people regarding condoms?

5 // Name one contraindication for using male condoms?

345   7 // Obstetrics And Gynaecology   The Unofficial Guide to Passing OSCEs: *Candidate Briefings, Patient Briefings and Mark Schemes*

O&G

# Station 9
## CERVICAL SMEAR COUNSELLING

*Candidate Briefing:* **Mrs Smith has arrived at your clinic after having a routine cervical smear. The result states she has moderate dyskaryosis. Please counsel her as to what this means and what options are available for management.**

*Patients Briefing:* **You are Mrs Smith, a 35 year old female who is attending clinic to discuss the result of your smear test.**

All your previous smears have been normal. You know the result is moderate dyskaryosis but you have no idea what this means. When asked about your concerns you are anxious to find out what happens next and you are concerned that it is cancer. (If the doctor does not ask about your concerns or does not address them within 2 minutes please blurt out 'it's cancer isn't it doctor', but be calmed once reassurance given.)

*If the doctor uses complicated, confusing medical language during their explanations appear confused, and if you are given the opportunity to ask questions ask them for clarification.*

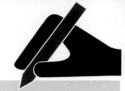

## Introduction

Clean hands, introduce self, confirm patient identity

Check identity of others in the room and confirm that the patient is happy for them to be present

Establish current patient knowledge and concerns

## Translation of Information

Explain what cervical smear screening is – specifically not looking for cancer, looking for early changes and treat if needed to stop cancer forming

Explain what patient's smear result means: abnormal smears common, not cancer, changes to the cervix that can happen for a number of reasons

Explain next advised step is colposcopy, and describe one

What might be done at colposcopy and why (biopsy/LLETZ)

Follow up: will contact you with date of colposcopy, will either require follow up smears or repeat colposcopy depending on what is done, will contact with results

Address concerns: no risk of passing it on through sex, does not affect fertility, advice stop smoking, and to avoid sex / swimming / tampons for two weeks post procedure

## Finishing the Consultation

Elicit patient concerns or questions

Summarise back to the patient

Arrange a follow up appointment (as necessary) or offer your contact details

Thank patient and close consultation

O&G

| Check patient understands regularly, and offer information leaflets | | | | |
|---|---|---|---|---|
| Maintain good eye contact and engage with patient | | | | |
| Avoid medical jargon | | | | |
| Polite to patient | | | | |

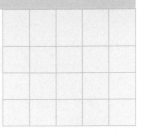

## Questions And Answers for Candidate

### What is the most common causes of cervical carcinoma and how is it acquired?

- HPV (Human papilloma virus) strains 16 and 18 acquired through sexual contact (not just intercourse)

### What is cervical excitation?

- The phenomenon whereby moving the cervix causes intense pain, this implies pelvic inflammation

O & G

1 // What age should women be offered cervical smears and how often?

2 // If severe dyskaryosis is found on the smear what is the next assessment that should be offered?

3 // State 2 treatment modalities for CIN.

4 // What staging system is used for cervical cancer?

# Chapter 8

# Psychiatry

*Candidate Briefing:* **Mr Chang is a 58-year-old man who has recently lost his job and has gone through a difficult divorce. Recent routine blood tests revealed an elevated GGT, and you are worried that this may be secondary to an alcohol problem. Please take a detailed alcohol history from him.**

*Patient Briefing:* **You are 58 years old and your name is Ivan Chang. Your wife left you 3 months ago. Since then you have increasingly been finding it hard to cope, turning to alcohol for comfort. You were a lawyer but recently lost your job as you kept turning up to work late looking dishevelled with several clients complaining about you. You are aware you have a problem, and desperately want help to take control of your life. You feel you are an embarrassment to your family who are now fed up with your behaviour and no longer contact you.**

Alcohol is always on your mind with much of your life dictated by it. You used to be quite social but comments from your friends about your alcohol intake angered you and you have found yourself spending much of your time at home drinking alone. You wake up craving for a drink and typically consume around 50 units a week mainly in the form of beers, with binge drinking up to 10 pints at a time, and drinking every day. This has increased significantly, with you needing more to have the same effect. You tried to stop drinking a month ago (for a week) but found yourself feeling very ill sweating and shaking. You restarted out of fear of feeling the same again. As of yet you have had no serious health complications from alcohol and suffer from no other medical or psychiatric conditions. You do not take any illicit drugs.

Your father was a heavy drinker and it led to significant problems in his marriage. You began drinking around 15 but have always been a social drinker up to now.

*You are aware of the dangers of drinking, seeing this in your father who was often hospitalised but know you need help to stop. You feel you may be depressed often feeling low in mood, tearful and lethargic. You wish to join a detox programme today.*

Psychiatry

## Mark Scheme for Examiner

### Introduction

| | | | | | |
|---|---|---|---|---|---|
| Clean hands, introduce self, confirm patient identity | | | | | |
| Explains purpose of consultation and obtain consent; collateral history if possible | | | | | |
| CAGE screening | | | | | |

### Alcohol Intake

| | | | | | |
|---|---|---|---|---|---|
| Daily/weekly intake (calculates units) | | | | | |
| Frequency of drinking/binge drinking | | | | | |
| Types of beverages | | | | | |
| Time of day starts drinking | | | | | |
| Drinking with company/alone | | | | | |

### Past Alcohol History

| | | | | | |
|---|---|---|---|---|---|
| Age started drinking and longest period of abstinence | | | | | |
| Family history of alcoholism | | | | | |
| Current or previous physical complications of alcohol usage | | | | | |
| Enquire about previous treatment e.g. detoxification programme / counselling | | | | | |

Psychiatry

## Screens for Alcohol Dependence Syndrome

| | | | | | |
|---|---|---|---|---|---|
| Compulsion | | | | | |
| Difficulties controlling intake | | | | | |
| Withdrawal and any health problems | | | | | |
| Tolerance | | | | | |
| Lack of other activities and interests | | | | | |
| Use despite harm | | | | | |

## Maintenance Factors

| | | | | | |
|---|---|---|---|---|---|
| Access to alcohol | | | | | |
| Triggers to start drinking | | | | | |

## Social Complications of Alcohol Abuse

| | | | | | |
|---|---|---|---|---|---|
| Job and relationship issues | | | | | |
| Criminal activity e.g. drink driving | | | | | |

## Risk assessment

| | | | | | |
|---|---|---|---|---|---|
| Screens for other substance misuse | | | | | |
| Screens for depression | | | | | |
| Insight (presence of illness, cause of illness, need for treatment) | | | | | |

## General Points

| | | | | | |
|---|---|---|---|---|---|
| Feedback on current intake and dangers of drinking | | | | | |
| Elicits patient concerns | | | | | |
| Summarises history back to patient | | | | | |

Psychiatry

| Explains help available and offer follow up | | | | | |
|---|---|---|---|---|---|
| Remains non-judgmental | | | | | |
| Responds to patient verbal and nonverbal cues | | | | | |
| Polite to patient | | | | | |
| Maintain good eye contact | | | | | |
| Appropriate use of open and closed questions | | | | | |
| Presentation of case | | | | | |

## Questions And Answers for Candidate

## How would you manage a case of alcohol withdrawal?

- For immediate relief you would give a benzodiazepine regime with doses calculated based on symptoms of withdrawal
- Pabrinex is also given over 3 days then thiamine (or vitamin B co-strong) is prescribed to supplement nutritional deficits
- The patient will require a more long term detoxification programme in the community and their GP should be contacted to help oversee this

## Describe three other pathological conditions linked strongly to excess alcohol consumption.

- Pancreatitis
- Hypertension
- Cardiac arrhythmias
- Iron deficiency anaemia
- GI bleeds, impaired clotting
- Cancer of the oropharynx, oesophagus, pancreas, liver and lungs
- Fetal alcohol syndrome
- Cerebellar degeneration and myopathy

Psychiatry

## What are the six key features of alcohol dependence syndrome?

- Strong desire or sense of compulsion to take the substance
- Difficulties controlling intake of the substance (either its onset, termination or levels of use)
- Physiological withdrawal state or the use of the same (or similar) substance to prevent such a withdrawal state: 'What happens when you stop drinking?'
- Tolerance (increasing amounts required to achieved desired effects): 'Are you finding yourself drinking more to get drunk?'
- Lack of other activities and interests
- Ongoing substance misuse despite clear evidence of harmful consequences

## Additional Questions to Consider

1 // **What are the recommended guidelines for alcohol consumption in one week for men and women?**

2 // **Why might an alcoholic be thiamine deficient? What symptoms does that present with?**

3 // **Describe the symptoms that might be experienced by a heavy alcohol user in withdrawal.**

4 // **What signs might you illicit when examining a chronic alcoholic?**

5 // **What is the mortality associated with acute delirium tremens?**

6 // **What public health interventions might be considered to reduce alcohol intake in society?**

Psychiatry

# Station 2
# DEPRESSION HISTORY

*Candidate Briefing:* **Mr Wood is a 50 year-old man who recently separated from his wife. His mood has been low and he has stopped caring about life. He has now lost his job. Please take a history from him and elicit any features of depression.**

*Patient Briefing:* **Your name is Sebastian Wood and you are 50 years old. Your wife left you 2 months ago, for another man. It was a complete shock to you and you haven't been coping without her in your life.**

3 weeks ago you lost your job as a car salesman, often turning up late to work and having sales at an all time low. You used to be very passionate about you work, and took great pride in your presentation. Now when you look in the mirror you don't recognise yourself. You have gone days without eating and stopped changing your clothes. Friends are concerned saying you've clearly lost weight (around 5kg) and never leave the house. Previously an active tennis player, now your energy levels are very low. You have lost interest in all your hobbies.

Your mood is low, particular first thing in the morning when you often feel tearful. Your sleep just isn't what it used to be. It takes ages for you to get to sleep and you seem to be awaking around 3am every day. You have very poor self-esteem. You feel worthless without your beloved Dianna around, and feel guilty you couldn't give her what she needed. It's very hard for you to concentrate when you try to watch television and you are beginning to forget important dates like your daughter's birthday last week.

*You have never had a manic episode and deny any psychotic symptoms. You have never had a psychiatric illness and prior to this were fit and well. You have never thought of harming yourself or ending your life. You don't want to go on feeling so low and welcome help. However you now live on your own without any close relationships.*

Psychiatry

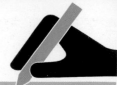

## Mark Scheme for Examiner

### Introduction

Introduce self

Identify patient (name, age, occupation)

Explains purpose of consultation and obtains consent

Collateral history if possible

### History

Duration of problem

### Core symptoms

Low mood, anhedonia, lack of energy

### Biological and Cognitive Symptoms

Enquire about sleep disturbance, appetite, weight loss, loss of libido, constipation

Enquire about worthlessness, self-esteem, poor memory / concentration, guilt, agitation

### Differential Diagnosis

Screens for mania and psychosis

Asks about medical problems (e.g. hypothyroidism), psychiatric problems, and current medication

### Risk Assessment

Suicide / self harm

Substance misuse

The Unofficial Guide to Passing OSCEs: *Candidate Briefings, Patient Briefings and Mark Schemes*

## Patient Beliefs

| | | | | | |
|---|---|---|---|---|---|
| Premorbid state | | | | | |
| Insight (awareness of illness, cause of illness and need for treatment) | | | | | |

## Social History

| | | | | | |
|---|---|---|---|---|---|
| Living and work circumstances | | | | | |
| Support network | | | | | |

## General Points

| | | | | | |
|---|---|---|---|---|---|
| Elicits patient concerns | | | | | |
| Summarises history back to patient | | | | | |
| Explains help available and offer follow up | | | | | |
| Remains non-judgmental | | | | | |
| Responds to patient verbal and nonverbal cues | | | | | |
| Polite to patient | | | | | |
| Maintain good eye contact | | | | | |
| Appropriate use of open and closed questions | | | | | |
| Presentation of case | | | | | |

---

### What are the three most alarming features of depression?

- Psychotic features
- Self neglect
- Potential for self harm / suicide

---

### What are the three core symptoms of depression?

- Low mood
- Low energy
- Loss of interest

---

### Give three examples of possible differential diagnosis for depression.

- Bipolar disorder
- Psychotic depression
- Drugs e.g. (alcohol, stimulant withdrawal, oral contraceptive pill, antihypertensive agents)
- Physical illness e.g. hypothyroidism
- Cushing's syndrome

1 // What are the benefits of using SSRIs in comparison to tricyclic antidepressants?

2 // When is electroconvulsive therapy indicated?

3 // Describe what social interventions you might suggest for a person suffering from depression.

4 // What other psychiatric disorders apart from depression can SSRIs be used for?

5 // How is clinical depression (or major depressive disorder) defined?

# Station 3
# MANIA COLLATERAL HISTORY

*Candidate Briefing:* **Mr Jones is worried about his wife. He reports that she has been acting out of sorts and has been on huge shopping sprees resulting in considerable debt. She often does not return home until the early hours of the morning. She has previously suffered from depression. Please take a history from her husband.**

*Patient Briefing:* **You have come in today as you are worried about your wife's recent change in behaviour.**

She is with you in the consultation. Normally quite sensible and the budgeter of the family, she has been on several shopping sprees resulting in considerable debt. She keeps coming back from work in the early hours of the morning and you worry she may get herself into trouble one of these days with neighbours complaining. You hardly see her sleep yet she says her energy levels and confidence have never been better. Every time you see her she seems to have taken up a new hobby. She is getting frustrated by your concern and doesn't want you to bring down her good mood. Her concentration is awful and she can't focus on one topic when you talk to her. She cannot understand why you think she is unwell.

**This has been going on for two weeks. You don't think she has any features of psychosis. She has not tried to harm herself or others. In the past she has battled with depression but is not currently on any medications.**

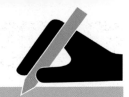

## Introduction

| | | | | | |
|---|---|---|---|---|---|
| Introduce self | | | | | |
| Establishes relationship of Mr Jones to patient | | | | | |
| Explains purpose of consultation and obtains consent | | | | | |

## History

| | | | | | |
|---|---|---|---|---|---|
| Enquires about recent stresses | | | | | |
| Duration of problem | | | | | |

## Symptoms of Manic Episode

| | | | | | |
|---|---|---|---|---|---|
| Mood | | | | | |
| Activity levels | | | | | |
| Disinhibition e.g. spending, increased sexual behaviour, trouble with the law | | | | | |
| Sleep pattern | | | | | |
| Confidence increased | | | | | |
| Concentration | | | | | |

## Differential Diagnosis

| | | | | | |
|---|---|---|---|---|---|
| Screens for psychosis | | | | | |
| Past medical history / drug history / psychiatric history | | | | | |

## Risk Assessment

| | | | | | |
|---|---|---|---|---|---|
| Suicide / self harm | | | | | |
| Substance misuse | | | | | |

Psychiatry

## General Questions

| | | | | | |
|---|---|---|---|---|---|
| Premorbid state | | | | | |
| Insight (awareness of illness, cause of illness and need for treatment) | | | | | |

## General Points

| | | | | | |
|---|---|---|---|---|---|
| Elicits patient concerns | | | | | |
| Summarises history back to patient | | | | | |
| Explains help available and offer follow up | | | | | |
| Remains non-judgmental | | | | | |
| Responds to patient verbal and nonverbal cues | | | | | |
| Polite to patient | | | | | |
| Maintain good eye contact | | | | | |
| Appropriate use of open and closed questions | | | | | |
| Presentation of case | | | | | |

## Questions And Answers for Candidate

### What is the difference between mania and hypomania?

- They are very similar and many of the same symptoms are experienced
- Hypomania isn't associated with psychotic symptoms, and is not severe enough to necessitate hospitalisation
- There is no significant impairment of day-to-day function, and it usually last for a less prolonged period

Psychiatry

## What is the definition of a manic episode?

A manic episode is a distinct period of persistently elevated, expansive and irritable mood. It must last for at least one week and features include:
- Inflated self-esteem or grandiosity
- Decreased need for sleep
- Talkative – more than usual
- Flight of ideas/racing thoughts
- Distractibility
- Increased goal-directed activity and psychomotor agitation
- Excessive involvement in pleasurable activities

## What is the difficulty when prescribing lithium and what are the signs and symptoms of overdose?

- Lithium has a very narrow therapeutic index. Toxicity can result in coarse tremor, nausea and vomiting, ataxia, confusion and cerebellar signs.

## Additional Questions to Consider

1 // What is the mean age of onset of bipolar affective disorder?

2 // In a patient presenting with a manic episode, what baseline investigations might you perform and why?

3 // What management options are there for bipolar affective disorder?

4 // Why may family therapy be important in the management of an individual suffering from bipolar affective disorder?

5 // What reversible causes might there be for mania?

# Station 4
## POST NATAL DEPRESSION

*Candidate Briefing:* **Mrs Roberts is a 24-year-old lady who has recently given birth to her first child. Her husband is concerned because Mrs Roberts doesn't appear to be coping well. Her mood has been persistently low and she has been very tearful. Please take a history from her.**

*Patient Briefing:* **You are Rachel Roberts. You are 24 years old and had your first baby girl Anabelle 1 week ago. Although the pregnancy was unexpected, your eventually grew fond of the idea with your husband standing by you throughout. The pregnancy was not complicated.**

You thought you'd feel happier when the baby arrived but instead you always feel on edge, worrying you can't look after her and that you're a bad mother. You feel you can't cope and had a baby too early in your life. You haven't been able to sleep properly since her arrival and feel guilty you are becoming so snappy to your husband. Breast feeding is a struggle. You don't have any other symptoms of depression, although you are very anxious.

**You have never had thoughts of harming Anabelle or yourself. There are no recent other life stresses you have encountered. You have never suffered from any psychiatric illnesses, and none run in the family. You have no medical illnesses, and you continue to have a very supportive husband.**

## Mark Scheme for Examiner

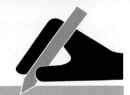

### Introduction

| | | | | |
|---|---|---|---|---|
| Introduce self | | | | |
| Identify patient | | | | |
| Explains purpose of consultation and obtains consent; collateral history if possible | | | | |

### History

| | | | | |
|---|---|---|---|---|
| Thoughts on pregnancy before birth | | | | |
| Enquires when gave birth | | | | |

### Symptoms of PND

| | | | | |
|---|---|---|---|---|
| Mood and symptoms of depression | | | | |
| Guilt / inadequacy towards baby / coping difficulties | | | | |
| Anxiety | | | | |
| Thoughts of harming the baby | | | | |
| Suicidal ideation | | | | |

### Screens Risk Factors

| | | | | |
|---|---|---|---|---|
| Person / family history of PND / depression | | | | |
| Poor social support / marital discord | | | | |
| Difficulties with breast feeding | | | | |
| Unplanned / unwanted pregnancy | | | | |
| Recent adverse life events | | | | |

Psychiatry

## Patient Beliefs

| | | | | | |
|---|---|---|---|---|---|
| Premorbid state | | | | | |
| Insight (awareness of illness, cause of illness and need for treatment) | | | | | |

## General Points

| | | | | | |
|---|---|---|---|---|---|
| Elicits patient concerns | | | | | |
| Summarises history back to patient | | | | | |
| Explains help available and offer follow up | | | | | |
| Remains non-judgmental | | | | | |
| Responds to patient verbal and nonverbal cues | | | | | |
| Polite to patient | | | | | |
| Maintain good eye contact | | | | | |
| Appropriate use of open and closed questions | | | | | |
| Presentation of case | | | | | |

## Questions And Answers for Candidate

### How would you manage a case of post natal depression?

- In mild cases guided self-help, exercise or watchful waiting; antidepressants and consideration of hospital admission only if severity warrants it

**What features does post natal depression have that differentiate it from a depressive episode?**

- High degree of anxiety
- Preoccupation with baby's health
- Feeling guilty about ability as a mother
- Reduced affection to the baby
- Obsessional phenomena regarding the baby
- Infanticidal thoughts and thoughts of harming the baby

**What cardiac complication is lithium therapy in pregnancy associated with?**

- Ebstein's anomaly

## Additional Questions to Consider

1 // Over what time period after birth can PND develop?

2 // When are you at higher risk of relapse into a pre-existing mental illness –in pregnancy or in the puerperium period and why?

3 // How does postnatal blues or "baby blues" present?

4 // What percentage of women suffer from postnatal blues?

5 // What are the differences between PND and puerperal psychosis?

Psychiatry

# Station 5
# SUICIDE RISK

*Candidate Briefing:* **James Smith is a 45-year-old recently separated gentleman who has attempted to hang himself. However, the rope gave way. He is now medically fit for psychiatric assessment and you are asked to see him. Take a history from him to establish his suicide risk.**

*Patient Briefing:* **Your name is James Smith. You are 45 years old and work as a mechanic. Your wife left you 3 weeks ago, taking with her your son (Rory 8 years old). Your marriage has not been the same since the death of your eldest (Francesca 12 years old) who was tragically abducted and killed. You were running late to pick her up from the park as you were out drinking with friends. Your wife blames you for the incident. She couldn't handle the constant arguments and decided it was best to leave and has had no contact since.**

You haven't been able to cope without them and no longer think life is worth living. For the past week you have been planning your suicide. One of your friends has moved in since the separation but you knew he would be away on a business trip today and therefore you wouldn't be found. You went out and bought some rope a week ago and keep it in the garage. You have written a note to your wife and your flatmate explaining why you can live no more, and left everything to your son in your will.

You drank a bottle of vodka in the lead up (and have been finding yourself drinking a lot more since the separation). You then attempted to hang yourself. However the rope gave way. Your flatmate came back early from his trip and was horrified to find you. You are upset you are still here and wish you had died. You don't see the point of this conversation. You do not want help and will try again to kill yourself. You have been depressed in the past but have never tried to harm yourself before and suffer from no major illnesses.

**You do not want to talk to your friends or wife about this. You have been feeling low for a while now and do not see a future or another way out of this situation. You have no real close relationships anymore. This is your first suicide attempt.**

The Unofficial Guide to Passing OSCEs: *Candidate Briefings, Patient Briefings and Mark Schemes*

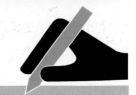

# Mark Scheme for Examiner

## Introduction

| | | | | | |
|---|---|---|---|---|---|
| Introduce self | | | | | |
| Identifies patient (name, age, occupation) | | | | | |
| Explains purpose of consultation and obtains consent; collateral history if possible | | | | | |

## Before the Suicide Attempt

| | | | | | |
|---|---|---|---|---|---|
| Recent stresses and trigger | | | | | |
| Planning | | | | | |
| Suicide notes / will | | | | | |
| Attempts to avoid detection | | | | | |

## Suicide Attempt

| | | | | | |
|---|---|---|---|---|---|
| Method | | | | | |
| Alcohol or drug use | | | | | |
| How was it discovered | | | | | |
| Potential fatality | | | | | |

## After Suicide Attempt

| | | | | | |
|---|---|---|---|---|---|
| Feelings about not being successful | | | | | |
| Thoughts about future | | | | | |
| Insight | | | | | |

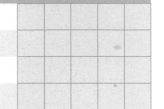
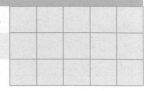

## Risk Factors

| | | | | | |
|---|---|---|---|---|---|
| Previous attempts / depression | | | | | |
| Support network: home circumstances, job circumstances, close confiding relationships | | | | | |
| Alcohol / drug abuse | | | | | |
| Sickness | | | | | |

## General Points

| | | | | | |
|---|---|---|---|---|---|
| Elicits patient concerns | | | | | |
| Summarises history back to patient | | | | | |
| Explains help available and offer follow up | | | | | |
| Remains non-judgmental | | | | | |
| Responds to patient verbal and nonverbal cues | | | | | |
| Polite to patient | | | | | |
| Maintain good eye contact | | | | | |
| Appropriate use of open and closed questions | | | | | |
| Presentation of case | | | | | |

## Questions And Answers for Candidate

### How might you deal with a low / medium risk suicide attempt in the community?

- Treat any underlying medical disease
- Challenge belief systems e.g. cognitive behavioural therapy
- Methods to reduce triggering factors e.g. work: reduced hours, less tight deadlines, relationships: referral to specialist groups such as 'Relate'

## Give four risk factors for completed suicide.

- Male gender
- Social class V, retired or unemployed, social isolation, divorced
- Previous deliberate self-harm, alcohol / drug abuse
- Physical illness
- Family history of psychiatric disorders, loss of rational thinking, age over 40 (or under 19)

## Which gender is deliberate self-harm most common in? Which gender is completed suicide more common it?

- Women are more likely than men to self-harm, but completed suicide is more likely in men

## Additional Questions to Consider

1 // State 3 psychiatric disorders associated with suicide.

2 // Discuss what population interventions could be carried out to help prevent suicide.

3 // If in your clinical history you find out that the individual has specific plans to harm another person, when would you consider breaking patient confidentiality and informing a third party?

4 // When would you consider detaining a patient who presented with suicidal ideation (i.e. in hospital, without their consent)?

5 // How would you differentiate a low, medium, and high risk suicide? What category would you put the above patient?

Psychiatry

# Station 6
# SCHIZOPHRENIA

*Candidate Briefing:* **Please take a history from this 19 year-old student, whose parents are worried is acting 'strange'. He has recently been hearing voices and believes his friends are out to get him.**

---

*Patient Briefing:* **Your name is Eric Smith. You are 19 years old and started university this year. Your parents have brought you to see the doctors today as they are worried about your 'strange' behaviour. You're not quite sure what they mean about this, but you have been having a tough time of late.**

Your classmates have all turned against you. Not only do they steal your thoughts in lectures leaving your mind blank but they also want to hurt you. You always feel afraid. They often whisper outside your door saying nasty things, but when you look there is no one there. The voices echo your thoughts. You don't know how, but they've even managed to send you threatening messages on the TV. You don't feel in control of your thoughts and worry others can hear them. You need someone to protect you from your classmates. You get upset if questioned about this not being true. The voices have never told you to harm yourself or others.

**You used a lot of cannabis at the start of university but otherwise have not had any psychiatric or medical problems. You have no thoughts of ending your life. You want to go back to how you were before university; a 'happy-go-lucky' guy with an active social life. Nowadays you spend much of your time alone in your room, but you don't have any symptoms of depression as such. However, you've started missing lectures to escape the threats.**

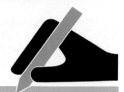

## Mark Scheme for Examiner

### Introduction

Introduce self

Identifies patient

Explains purpose of consultation and obtains consent; collateral history if possible

### Delusions

Screens for at least 3 delusion types e.g. persecutory, delusions of reference, grandeur, nihilistic

Test conviction

Assesses passivity / Feeling of loss of control

### Auditory Hallucinations

Content: any thought echo

Third person / Second person

Instructions to harm yourself or others

Screens for other hallucinations e.g. visual / olfactory / gustatory

### Thought Interference

Thought insertion

Thought withdrawal

Thought broadcast

## Differential Diagnosis

| | | | | | |
|---|---|---|---|---|---|
| Recent drug / alcohol use | | | | | |
| Mood – low / elated in the past | | | | | |
| Health problems: medical, psychiatric, (including family history), current medications | | | | | |

## Patient Beliefs

| | | | | | |
|---|---|---|---|---|---|
| Premorbid personality | | | | | |
| Insight (presence of illness, cause of illness, need for treatment) | | | | | |

## Social History

| | | | | | |
|---|---|---|---|---|---|
| Support network: home circumstances, job circumstances, relationships | | | | | |
| Current stresses | | | | | |

## General Points

| | | | | | |
|---|---|---|---|---|---|
| Elicits patient concerns | | | | | |
| Summarises history back to patient | | | | | |
| Explains help available and offer follow up | | | | | |
| Remains non-judgmental | | | | | |
| Responds to patient verbal and nonverbal cues | | | | | |
| Polite to patient | | | | | |
| Maintain good eye contact | | | | | |
| Appropriate use of open and closed questions | | | | | |
| Presentation of case | | | | | |

### Define delusion, hallucination, and psychosis.

- Delusion: fixed false belief which is not congruent with cultural norms
- Hallucination: perception in the absence of a stimulus
- Psychosis: loss of contact with reality

### What are the typical hallucinations associated with Schizophrenia?

- Third person auditory halluncinations

1 // What do the terms positive and negative symptoms mean in relation to schizophrenia?

2 // What side effects are particularly problematic in typical antipsychotics?

3 // Why is olanzapine not first-line for a patient with type 1 diabetes mellitus?

4 // Why is clozapine less likely to be used in schizophrenia, except in treatment-resistant cases?

5 // How would you manage a patient with schizophrenia?

*Candidate Briefing:* **Mrs Bradley has recently separated from her husband, and lost her job. She seems to be very depressed. Please perform a mental state examination on her and present your findings.**

*Patient Briefing:* **Your name is Samantha Bradley. You are 56 years old. Your husband left you 2 weeks ago and you have been feeling very down since. You used to work in the laundrette but were sacked for persistent tardiness.**

**Appearance and behaviour:** You remain well kempt and generally look in good health. You are able to engage with the doctor and maintain eye contact but do become rather tearful when asked about your husband.

**Mood:** Your mood is very low and you are aware of this. You've noticed is varies a lot in the day. You deny ever feeling elated or having suicidal ideation.

**Speech:** Normal tone, rhythm, rate and volume

**Thoughts:** You have no problem processing your thoughts and are able to have a clear conversation with the doctor. You are aware that for the past 2 weeks your thoughts have been preoccupied with thoughts of your husband. You still can't believe he left you. He said to you he wanted a fresh go at life. He felt your relationship had become dull and neither of you could be the best you could possibly be while you were still together. Either he was having a mid life crisis or he was hiding an affair. You just didn't quite buy his explanation but he has not contacted you since. You deny self harm thoughts or abnormal thoughts.

**Perceptions:** No abnormal perceptions

**Cognition:** You are orientated in time, place and person. You are able to perform serial 7s.

*Insight: You know your low mood is a consequence of your husband leaving you and would welcome any treatment offered.*

Psychiatry

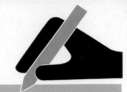

## Introduction

Introduce self (wash hands before touching patient)

Identify patient

Explains purpose of consultation and obtain consent

## Appearance and Behaviour

Dress

Evidence of self-harm

Evidence of physical neglect

Evidence of physical illness

Quality of rapport and eye contact

Tearful / anxious / suspicious

## Mood

Screens for depression

Screens for mania

Affect

Suicidal ideations and harming

## Speech

Tone

Rhythm

Rate

Volume

Psychiatry

## Thoughts

| | | | | | |
|---|---|---|---|---|---|
| Coherence of conversation (thought form disorder) | | | | | |
| Worries / preoccupations / obsessional ruminations | | | | | |
| Self harm thoughts | | | | | |
| Screens for psychosis | | | | | |

## Perception

| | | | | | |
|---|---|---|---|---|---|
| Hallucinations (particularly auditory) | | | | | |

## Cognition

| | | | | | |
|---|---|---|---|---|---|
| Orientation in time, place and person | | | | | |
| Concentration: Serials 7s / months in reverse order | | | | | |

## Insight

| | | | | | |
|---|---|---|---|---|---|
| Insight into illness (cause of illness, presence of illness, need for treatment) | | | | | |

## General Points

| | | | | | |
|---|---|---|---|---|---|
| Elicits patient concerns | | | | | |
| Summarises history back to patient | | | | | |
| Explains help available and offer follow up | | | | | |
| Remains non-judgmental | | | | | |
| Responds to patient verbal and nonverbal cues | | | | | |
| Polite to patient | | | | | |
| Maintain good eye contact | | | | | |
| Appropriate use of open and closed questions | | | | | |
| Presentation of case | | | | | |

Psychiatry

---

### How do you classify hallucinations? What is the benefit of classification?

- Hallucinations can be 1st person, 2nd person or 3rd person
- They can be auditory, visual, tactile, olfactory or gustatory
- This helps point to a diagnosis, for example, third person auditory hallucinations are classically associated with schizophrenia

---

### Describe how you go about assessing insight. What aspects of the illness would you seek to assess patient insight into?

- Take a history, speak to the patient about their illness: Is the patient aware of their illness? Is the patient aware of the cause of their illness? Is the patient aware of the need for treatment?

---

### What is the difference between thought form and thought content?

- Thought form is the 'mechanics' of thinking, i.e. how thoughts are organised, and how one idea is connected to the next idea in the patient's head. If there is disturbance in the logical connection between ideas, a thought form disorder might be present. An example of this is 'knights move thinking' when a person jumps from one idea to something completely unrelated.
- Thought content is 'the what' of thought i.e. the beliefs (content of thought) held by the patient e.g. suicidal ideation.

Psychiatry

1 // What is pressured speech?

2 // Give some examples of abnormalities in thought form.

3 // How might the appearance of a patient suggest a manic episode?

4 // How might the speech of a patient suggest a depressive episode?

5 // How would you manage a case of severe depression?

Psychiatry

# Station 8
## COGNITIVE EXAMINATION

*Candidate Briefing:* **Mr Ahmed is a 68 year-old man who has been referred because his son has noticed his increasing forgetfulness. The son worries that his father may have some memory problems. Please make an assessment of the father's mental state.**

*Patient Briefing:* **Your name is Mohammed Ahmed. You are 68 years old and are a retired school teacher. Your son has brought you to the GP today as he has increasing concerns about your forgetfulness.**

You feel guilty you are causing so much concern but aren't sure what all the fuss is about. Sure your memory isn't what it used to be, but isn't that just a part of getting older? You can't pinpoint when this started so assume it has been a gradual thing. You have difficulties with remembering important dates and are very annoyed you recently forgot your grandson birthday. You have found yourself increasingly getting lost in familiar places. Last week a neighbour found you wandering in the street as you had forgotten where your house was. She has also expressed concerns over your safety.

*When the doctor performs the assessment, you will give the following mixture of correct and incorrect answers:*

**Orientation:** Not orientated in time (0/5), able to name country but otherwise not orientated in place (1/5)
**Registration:** register all three items (3/3)
**Attention and calculation:** (3/5) D-L –O-R-W
**Recall:** (0/3) No objects remembered
**Language:** (3/3) Able to name pen and watch. Can repeat sentence.
**Reading and writing:** (2/2) Reads and follows command.
Writes 'Good luck with your OSCEs.'
**Three stage command:** (2/3) Forgets to place paper on floor but otherwise successful.
**Construction:** (1/1) Copies successfully
MMSE score 15/30

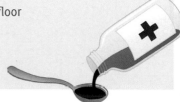

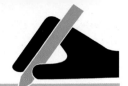

# Mark Scheme for Examiner

## Introduction

Introduce self

Identify patient

Explains purpose of consultation and obtain consent

## History

Establishes nature of problem, including collateral history if possible

Duration

Affect on life

## Orientation

Date, day, month, year, season

## Place

Country, county, town / city, building name, floor

## Registration

Say 3 common objects and give 1 point per word remembered; can repeat up to 6 times until all 3 remembered but record trails

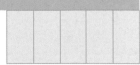

## Attention and Calculation

Subtract 7 from 100. 1 point for each correct answer

| | | | | |
|---|---|---|---|---|
| | | | | |

Stop after 5 answers (93, 86, 79, 72, 65)

| | | | | |
|---|---|---|---|---|
| | | | | |

Or WORLD backwards. 1 point for each correct letter
D-L-R-O-W

| | | | | |
|---|---|---|---|---|
| | | | | |

## Recall

1 point per word remembered

| | | | | |
|---|---|---|---|---|
| | | | | |

## Language

Recognises watch and pen when pointed to

| | | |
|---|---|---|
| | | |

Repeats 'No ifs, ands or buts'

| | | |
|---|---|---|
| | | |

## Reading and Writing

Reads 'close your eyes' and follows command

| | | |
|---|---|---|
| | | |

## Three stage Command

1 point per command performed. Do not mime or demonstrate the command

| | | | |
|---|---|---|---|
| | | | |

## Construction

Score 1 if each pentagon has 5 sides and there is a diamond shape in the middle; if there are any errors, then the patient scores 0

| | | |
|---|---|---|
| | | |

## General Points

Accurately calculates MMSE score out of 30

| | | |
|---|---|---|
| | | |

Interprets score

| | | |
|---|---|---|
| | | |

Explains help available and offer follow up

| | | |
|---|---|---|
| | | |

Psychiatry

| Remains non-judgmental | | | | |
|---|---|---|---|---|
| Responds to patient verbal and nonverbal cues | | | | |
| Polite to patient | | | | |
| Maintain good eye contact | | | | |

## What chromosomal abnormality is associated with early onset dementia?

- Down syndrome (Trisomy 21)

## Name three different causes of dementia.

- Alzheimers Disease
- Lewy Body Dementia
- Frontotemperal Dementia
- Vascular Dementia
- Wilson's Disease

1 // How would you interpret this score? What is your differential diagnosis?

2 // What investigations might you perform in a new diagnosis of dementia?

3 // How would you differentiate a delirium from a dementia?

4 // What treatment options are available for dementia?

5 // What is Lewy body dementia? How is this differentiated from other forms of dementia?

# Chapter 9

# Paediatrics

# Station 1
# THE CRYING BABY

*Candidate Briefing: Mrs Jones is a 32 year-old mother of Mabel who is 5 months old. She is consulting her GP today as Mabel will not stop crying. Please take a full history from Mrs Jones about her child.*

*Patient Briefing: You are Mrs Jones, Mabel's mum. Mabel has had occasional intermittent crying since birth lasting up to 1 hour. It often follows feeding and can be associated with small vomits. Today the crying is more persistent, and is not just related to feeds. It is not high pitched. Nothing seems to help. She also has a fever, a cough and a runny nose. She has been rubbing her right ear a lot.*

Mabel's birth and past medical history are unremarkable. She is breast fed and feeds well. Her weight is on the 50th centile. You live at home with Mabel and Mabel's father. You have coped well as a family with the crying until this point.

*Your main concern is that today's episode is unusual for her and you are worried she may be very unwell with an infection.*

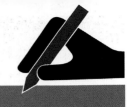

## Mark Scheme for Examiner

## Introduction

| | | | | |
|---|---|---|---|---|
| Clean hands, introduce self, confirm patient identity (and relationship of any other present), and gain consent for history taking | | | | |

## Presenting Complaint (crying)

| | | | | |
|---|---|---|---|---|
| Onset (gradual/sudden) | ✓ | | | |
| Frequency | ✓ | | | |
| Duration (of each episode, and of crying in general) | ✓ | | | |
| Intermittent or constant | ✓ | | | |
| Character (e.g. high pitched) | | | | |
| Triggers (e.g. introduction of milk) | | | | |
| Timing (in relation to feeds/time of day) | ✓ | | | |
| Has anything helped (e.g. posture, and are they consolable) | | | | |
| What makes it worse (e.g. feeding) | | | | |
| Associated symptoms/systemic enquiry (e.g. fever, rashes, drawing up of knees, rashes, back arching) | ✓ | | | |

## Past Medical History

| | | | | |
|---|---|---|---|---|
| Antenatal history | ✓ | | | |
| Birth history (gestation, delivery method, intensive care admission) | ✓ | | | |
| Previous hospital admissions, and long term medical problems being followed up in the community / hospital (including investigations) | | | | |

Paediatrics

## Drug History

| Drug and allergy history, immunisations | ✓ | | | | |
|---|---|---|---|---|---|

## Growth and Development

| Height and weight centiles (current, and whether following centile lines) | ✓ | | | | |
|---|---|---|---|---|---|
| Developmental milestones (gross motor, fine motor, social, vision and hearing) | ✓ | | | | |

## Nutritional History

| Current feeding (method and frequency, compared to normal) | ✓ | | | | |
|---|---|---|---|---|---|
| Number of wet and dirty nappies (compared to normal) | ✓ | | | | |

## Family History

| Family history | ✓ | | | | |
|---|---|---|---|---|---|

## Social History

| Family tree (including age and who lives at home) | ✓ | | | | |
|---|---|---|---|---|---|
| Home environment (inc smoking/pets) | ✓ | | | | |
| Recent travel | ✓ | | | | |

## Finishing the Consultation

| Elicit parent concerns and impact of crying on family | | | | | |
|---|---|---|---|---|---|
| Summarise history back to parent | ✓ | | | | |
| Thank parent and close consultation | ✓ | | | | |

Paediatrics

## General Points

| Polite to patient | ✓ | | | |
|---|---|---|---|---|
| Maintain good eye contact | / | | | |
| Appropriate use of open and closed questions | / | | | |
| Presentation of case | / | | | |

## Questions And Answers for Candidate

### If the crying was high pitched, name two diagnoses you may be concerned about.

- Meningitis/infection
- Intracranial bleed
- Drug withdrawal/birth asphyxia (in a newborn baby)
- Genetic syndromes e.g. cri du chat

### In what ways could you initially manage gastroeosophageal reflux in a baby?

- Initially positional advice can be used, particularly in younger babies: feeding the baby in a more upright position, and keeping the baby upright for about 20 minutes after feeds
- In addition, at night the head of the moses basket (if they are still in one) could be tilted up
- Medical treatment with domperidone, or ranitidine could be considered, as well as feed thickeners or gaviscon therapy

> **If you were concerned about an intussusception, which imaging test would be most appropriate?**

- Ultrasound of abdomen

> **How would you manage bronchiolitis?**

- The management consists of respiratory and feeding support
- Breathing: supplementary oxygen if low saturations; may require CPAP or intubation
- Feeding: if not feeding adequately, attempt reducing feed frequency and volume; if this is not effective, consider NG feeding or IV fluids

# ? Additional Questions to Consider

**1 //** How do you treat intussusception?

**2 //** What risk factors might predispose this child to have bronchiolitis?

**3 //** What makes babies more susceptible to reflux?

**4 //** If you found evidence of a hernia, how would differentiate between it being obstructed and non obstructed on examination?

**5 //** How would you manage suspected meningitis in a baby?

Paediatrics

# Station 2
# FEBRILE CONVULSIONS

*Candidate Briefing: You are asked to see Fred, a 2 year-old child who has been brought in with his mother. He has presented with a temperature and a fit. You examined the patient and found signs consistent with acute otitis media. Take a history from the mother and suggest a possible diagnosis.*

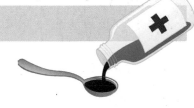

*Patient Briefing: You are Fred's mother. You come into hospital with your only child, Fred. He had a 5 minute fit at home today that ended by itself. He was completely fine beforehand, other than tugging at his ear, and feeling hot. The fit involved the whole of his body shaking and then going floppy. He fully recovered within five minutes. You are very concerned since you brother has serious epilepsy, having to go to intensive care on two occasions with prolonged fits.*

Fred was a term baby, with no medical problems, and no admissions to hospital except an overnight admission with pneumonia last year. He is growing well, meeting his developmental milestones. Feeding is normal.

*You live at home with Fred and your husband.*

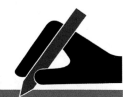

## Mark Scheme for Examiner

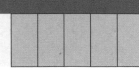

## Introduction

| Clean hands, introduce self (to parent and child), confirm patient and parent identity (and relationship of any other present), and gain consent for history taking | | | | | |
|---|---|---|---|---|---|

Paediatrics

## Presenting Complaint

| | | | | | |
|---|---|---|---|---|---|
| Pre-fit state | | | | | |
| Any temperature? If so enquire about a focus | | | | | |
| Length of fit | | | | | |
| Description of fit (including symmetry of movement, colour change, loss of consciousness, injuries sustained) | | | | | |
| Post-fit state (specifically ask about length of time to recover) | | | | | |
| Is recovery complete? Any residual weakness? | | | | | |

## Past Medical History

| | | | | | |
|---|---|---|---|---|---|
| Antenatal history | | | | | |
| Birth history (gestation, delivery method, intensive care admission) | | | | | |
| Previous hospital admissions, and long term medical problems being followed up in the community/hospital (including investigations) | | | | | |
| Ask specifically about epilepsy / febrile convulsions | | | | | |

## Drug History

| | | | | | |
|---|---|---|---|---|---|
| Drug and allergy history, immunisations | | | | | |

## Growth and Development

| | | | | | |
|---|---|---|---|---|---|
| Height and weight centiles (current, and whether following centile lines) | | | | | |
| Developmental milestones (gross motor, fine motor, social, vision and hearing) | | | | | |

Paediatrics

## Nutritional History

| | | | | | |
|---|---|---|---|---|---|
| Current feeding (method and frequency, compared to normal) | | | | | |
| Urine and stool (compared to normal) | | | | | |

## Family History

| | | | | | |
|---|---|---|---|---|---|
| Family history (including epilepsy and febrile convulsions) | | | | | |

## Social History

| | | | | | |
|---|---|---|---|---|---|
| Family tree (including age and who lives at home) | | | | | |
| Home environment (inc smoking/pets) | | | | | |
| Recent travel | | | | | |

## Finishing the Consultation

| | | | | | |
|---|---|---|---|---|---|
| Elicit parent concerns and impact of crying on family | | | | | |
| Summarise history back to parent | | | | | |
| Thank parent and close consultation | | | | | |

## General Points

| | | | | | |
|---|---|---|---|---|---|
| Polite to patient | | | | | |
| Maintain good eye contact | | | | | |
| Appropriate use of open and closed questions | | | | | |
| Presentation of case | | | | | |

### What is the typical age range for febrile convulsions?

- Six months to six years

### What is the long term prognosis for someone with a febrile convulsion?

- Children tend to grow out of febrile convulsions, and develop normally
- For simple febrile convulsions, the increased risk of developing epilepsy is small compared to the risk in the general population

### How do you treat a febrile convulsion?

- Convulsions should be managed as per any seizure, with consideration of benzodiazepines first to halt a prolonged seizure
- Febrile convulsions usually stop without the need for any intervention
- Any source of fever e.g. otitis media should be treated
- Antipyretics should be considered for when the patient has any subsequent temperature
- The patient should be advised to return to hospital if they have another febrile convulsion during the same illness

Paediatrics

**1 //** How common are febrile convulsions?

**2 //** What is a breath holding attack?

**3 //** What would make you worry that the seizure was due to space occupying legion?

**4 //** How do you differentiate a rigor from a seizure?

**5 //** How long does a febrile convulsion typical last for?

# Station 3
# WHEEZE

*Candidate Briefing: Tommy, a 3 year-old boy, has presented to the Accident and Emergency department with wheeze. Please take a history from Mrs McShire, his mother.*

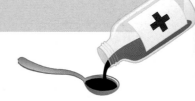

*Patient Briefing: You are the mother of Tommy a 3 year old boy, who has been wheezy today and breathless. It is getting progressively worse: he is now constantly wheezy and breathless. You have tried using your older child's asthma inhaler, which helped a little bit but wore off quickly. You can't think of any obvious triggers, but Tommy has had a runny nose, and a cough for the last 2 days.*

Tommy was born on time, and has had no medical problems, except eczema, which is managed by the GP. He is otherwise well with no exercise limitation, or cough at night. He is on no medications, has no allergies and immunisations are up to date. He is growing well, following the 50th centile for height and weight. Other than his brother having asthma, there is no significant family history. Both you and your husband smoke 20 cigarettes a day. You live in a two bedroom flat with your two children, and don't have any pets.

*You are really worried that this might be asthma.*

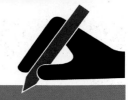

## Mark Scheme for Examiner

### Introduction

Clean hands, introduce self (to parent and child), confirm patient and parent identity (and relationship of any other present), and gain consent for history taking

### Presenting Complaint

Clarify what parents mean by wheeze

Onset (time, gradual/sudden)

Progress (getting worse/better)

Constant or intermittent

Degree of breathlessness

How was he pre-wheezing? Any triggers?

Any interventions tried?

### Past Medical History

Birth history (gestation, delivery method, intensive care admission)

Previous hospital admissions, and long term medical problems being followed up in the community/hospital (including investigation)

Ask specifically about bronchiolitis, viral induced wheeze, asthma, eczema, allergy

Interval symptoms (nocturnal cough, exercise limitation)

### Drug History

Drug and allergy history, recent courses of steroids, immunisations

Paediatrics

## Growth and Development

| | | | | | |
|---|---|---|---|---|---|
| Height and weight centiles (current, and whether following centile lines) | | | | | |
| Developmental milestones (gross motor, fine motor, social, vision and hearing) | | | | | |

## Nutritional History

| | | | | | |
|---|---|---|---|---|---|
| Current feeding (method and frequency, compared to normal) | | | | | |
| Urine and stool (compared to normal) | | | | | |

## Family History

| | | | | | |
|---|---|---|---|---|---|
| Family history (including asthma, eczema, atopy) | | | | | |

## Social History

| | | | | | |
|---|---|---|---|---|---|
| Family tree (including age and who lives at home) | | | | | |
| Home environment (inc smoking/pets, recent change of address) | | | | | |
| Recent travel | | | | | |

## Finishing the Consultation

| | | | | | |
|---|---|---|---|---|---|
| Elicit parent concerns and impact of crying on family | | | | | |
| Summarise history back to parent | | | | | |
| Thank parent and close consultation | | | | | |

Paediatrics

The Unofficial Guide to Passing OSCEs: *Candidate Briefings, Patient Briefings and Mark Schemes*

## General Points

| | | | | |
|---|---|---|---|---|
| Polite to patient | | | | |
| Maintain good eye contact | | | | |
| Appropriate use of open and closed questions | | | | |
| Presentation of case | | | | |

## Questions And Answers for Candidate

### Give three possible causes of wheeze in a child.

- Anaphalaxis
- Viral induced wheeze
- Asthma
- Bronchiolitis
- Inhaled foreign body
- Heart failure
- Gastro-oesophageal reflux

### What additional diseases might be associated with asthma, either in the child or in the family?

- Eczema
- Hayfever
- Allergies
- Asthma (in the family)
- Cow's milk protein intolerance

> **Is the child still at risk of worsening respiratory symptoms if the parents only smoke outside?**
>
> - Yes: harmful substances from smoke remain on the parent's clothes, and breath
> - The advice should be that the parents give up smoking completely

 **Additional Questions to Consider**

1 // Give three indications of a life threatening exacerbation of asthma.

2 // Give three indications of a severe exacerbation of asthma.

3 // What environmental triggers do you know that might trigger an asthma exacerbation?

4 // What would you do for an asthmatic 3 year old child who is not being adequately controlled in the community on a salbutamol inhaler?

5 // How would you differentiate asthma from a viral induced wheeze?

# Station 4
# DIABETES MELLITUS (TYPE 1)

*Candidate Briefing: Zac White is a 14 year-old boy who has been recently diagnosed with diabetes and is about to commence insulin therapy. Please explain the diagnosis, and options for insulin treatment to him. Address any concerns he and his parents may have.*

*Patient Briefing: You are Zac, and have just attended A/E, with drinking more, peeing more, and losing weight. You have been diagnosed as having type 1 diabetes, and a doctor has come to you to explain the diagnosis and the treatment which is about to be commenced. Mum is with you, but you speak to the doctor directly.*

You have a good understanding of what diabetes is, and that you need to start insulin. However you are really worried about what happens when your sugar levels drop, and think you could die from low sugars.

*This is making you very anxious, and you seek reassurance from the doctor. You are also anxious because your uncle with type II diabetes died of a heart attack that the doctors said was related to his diabetes.*

## Mark Scheme for Examiner

## Introduction

| | | | | | |
|---|---|---|---|---|---|
| Cleans hands, introduces self, confirms patient identity | | | | | |
| Check identity of others in the room and confirm that the patient is happy for them to be present | | | | | |
| Establish current patient knowledge and concerns | | | | | |

## Explain Diabetes

| | | | | | |
|---|---|---|---|---|---|
| Explain the cause of diabetes, and why it is treated | | | | | |

## Explain Insulin Therapy

| | | | | | |
|---|---|---|---|---|---|
| Explain about the need for injecting insulin | | | | | |
| Explain about the 'basal bolus' regime, and potential other options | | | | | |
| Mention rotating injection site and the reason behind this | | | | | |

## Explain Complication of Diabetes

| | | | | | |
|---|---|---|---|---|---|
| Explain about low sugar levels, the need to monitor sugar levels, and how it might be recognised | | | | | |
| Explain about when to treat low sugar levels | | | | | |
| Explain about long term, multidisciplinary follow up to ensure good sugar control, and identify any potential complications early | | | | | |

Paediatrics

## Finishing the Consultation

| | | | | | |
|---|---|---|---|---|---|
| Elicit patient concerns or questions | | | | | |
| Summarise history back to parent | | | | | |
| Arrange a follow up appointment, offer your contact details, provide written information | | | | | |
| Thank parent and close consultation | | | | | |

## General Points

| | | | | | |
|---|---|---|---|---|---|
| Check patient understands regularly, and offer information leaflets | | | | | |
| Maintain good eye contact | | | | | |
| Avoid medical jargon | | | | | |
| Polite to patient | | | | | |

## Questions And Answers for Candidate

### What might cause a patient to present in DKA (2 examples)?

- New diagnosis of diabetes
- Infection
- Poor compliance with medication
- Myocardial infarction (older patients)

What antibodies might be worth testing for in a new diagnosis of suspected type 1 diabetes?

- Anti-Islet cell antibodies
- Anti-GAD antibodies

What are the classic presenting symptoms of type 1 diabetics?

- Polyuria
- Polydipsia
- Weight loss
- Polyphagia

# ? Additional Questions to Consider

1 // What other autoimmune diseases are associated with type 1 diabetes?

2 // What are the main complications of type 1 diabetes?

3 // What is HBA1c? What would be a good target to aim for to indicate well controlled diabetes?

4 // What are the advantages and disadvantages of using an insulin pump?

5 // How will having diabetes affect driving in the future?

*Candidate Briefing: Ahmed, a 5 month-old baby boy, has been brought to the Emergency Department by his mother after he "rolled off the sofa". He has broken his right humerus. You are asked to see his mother in the ED about his injury.*

*Patient Briefing: You are the mother of a five month old boy Ahmed, and have arrived in the emergency department. 4 days ago you came home to find him in pain. He had been looked after by your brother that day. You do not know exactly what happened, but your brother had said Ahmed 'rolled off the sofa' and that there was no need to get him checked out. You have never seen him roll before, and are a little bit suspicious of the story, but give your brother the benefit of the doubt. However, four days later Ahmed still seems to be in pain so you come to the emergency department to get him checked out.*

You are a single parent, and have no contact with Ahmed's father. Your brother has been increasingly helping out at home, but he is occasionally aggressive and violent towards you. You don't want him to get into trouble, as he has been in trouble with the law before, so you instead say that you saw Ahmed roll off the sofa, not him.

Life is becoming more of a struggle and you have resorted to alcohol.

You do not have a social worker.

Ahmed was born on time, and has had no medical problems before. He is small for his age, but developing normally. You also have a 3 year old daughter. She has been to the emergency department three times in the last 3 months with injuries.

*When questioned, you get anxious and aggressive about whether he has rolled over in the past. You will volunteer your concerns about your brother only if the doctor remains non judgemental and caring throughout the consultation.*

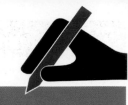

# Mark Scheme for Examiner

## Introduction

Clean hands, introduce self (to parent and child), confirm patient and parent identity (and relationship of any other present), and gain consent for history taking

## Presenting Complaint

Obtain a clear account of the events that occurred leading up to the injury

Note the time of injury and any delay in presentation

Ask about any witnesses to the event

Get third party accounts of the events if possible

## Past Medical History

Birth history (gestation, delivery method, intensive care admission)

Previous hospital admissions (including which hospitals attended), and any long term medical problems

## Drug History

Drug and allergy history, immunisations

## Growth and Development

Height and weight centiles (current, and whether following centile lines)

Developmental milestones (gross motor, fine motor, social, vision and hearing)

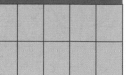

Paediatrics

## Nutritional History

| | | | | |
|---|---|---|---|---|
| Current feeding (method and frequency, compared to normal) | | | | |
| Number of wet and dirty nappies (compared to normal) | | | | |

## Family History

| | | | | |
|---|---|---|---|---|
| Family history | | | | |

## Social History

| | | | | |
|---|---|---|---|---|
| Home environment: who is at home (parents, siblings, other), any current coping issues | | | | |
| Drug/alcohol problems, criminal records, medical / psychological illness in parents | | | | |
| Any current involvement with social services (relating to this child, other children, or the parents) | | | | |
| Family tree (including age and who lives at home) | | | | |

## Finishing the Consultation

| | | | | |
|---|---|---|---|---|
| Elicit parent concerns and impact on family | | | | |
| Summarise history back to parent | | | | |
| Thank parent and close consultation | | | | |

## General Points

| | | | | |
|---|---|---|---|---|
| Remain calm and non judgmental | | | | |
| Avoid leading questions | | | | |
| Polite to patient | | | | |
| Maintain good eye contact | | | | |
| Appropriate use of open and closed questions | | | | |
| Presentation of case | | | | |

Paediatrics

**What investigations might be considered in a suspected case of non accidental injury (four)?**

- Bloods (FBC / clotting),  skeletal survey, CT head, ophthalmological assessment
- Also consider: STI screen (sexual abuse), ultrasound (tissue haematoma), dentist review (bite marks), plastic surgery review (burns)

**What are the four broad domains than can be used to categorize child abuse?**

- Physical: causing physical harm
- Emotional: constant neglect or ill treatment, adversely affecting emotional development
- Neglect: constant failure to meet basic needs of the child
- Sexual: enforcing / enticing sexual activity, including non penetrative acts

**What is a spiral fracture, and what type of injury is it associated with?**

- A fracture where at least one part of the bone has been twisted; the fracture line is helical and usually results from a twisting injury

**1 //**   What in the history might make you worry about NAI?

**2 //**   How would you differentiate between suspicious and non suspicious bruising?

**3 //**   What is a skeletal survey?

**4 //**   What are the causes of petechiae in a child?

**5 //**   What fracture pattern would make you worry about NAI?

*Candidate Briefing: Mr and Mrs Fletcher have come to your clinic with their son Sandy. They are keen to get the MMR vaccine for him, but have some concerns about what they have heard in the media. Please discuss the pros and cons of getting the MMR vaccine with his parents.*

*Patient Briefing: You are the dad of Sandy, an 11 month old baby. You would like to discuss the MMR vaccine, but know little about it. Sandy is currently fit and well, with no medical problems. You have read about the link between the vaccine and autism, and this is the biggest thing worrying you.*

## Mark Scheme for Examiner

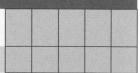

### Introduction

| | | | | |
|---|---|---|---|---|
| Clean hands, introduce self (to parent and child), confirm patient and parent identity | | | | |
| Check identity of others in the room and confirm that the patient is happy for them to be present | | | | |
| Establish current patient knowledge and concerns | | | | |

### Explaining the Vaccine

| | | | | |
|---|---|---|---|---|
| Explains what the vaccine is, when it's given, and the benefits to the child of taking it | | | | |
| Explains herd immunity benefit | | | | |

### Explain the Contraindications

| | | | | |
|---|---|---|---|---|
| Immunocompromised, malignancy, another live vaccine in previous three years, acute febrile illness, allergies to gelatine or neomycin | | | | |

Paediatrics

## Explains Risks

Fever or rash within one week of immunisation

No evidence of link to autism, or inflammatory bowel disease

## Explains Alternatives

Single jab: six injections instead of two, longer time to full immunisation, poor compliance possibility, more painful / traumatic to the child

## Finishing the Consultation

Elicit patient concerns or questions

Summarise back to the patient

Arrange a follow up appointment (as necessary) or offer your contact details

Thank parent and close consultation

## General Points

Check patient understands regularly, and offer information leaflets

Maintain good eye contact and engage with patient

Avoid medical jargon

Polite to patient

---

### What are the disadvantages of single vaccines instead of MMR?

- Requires 6 jabs instead of 2: more pain to child, and may result in poorer compliance due to number of visits required
- The child is fully immunized later: therefore more vulnerable to infection for longer

---

### What is the link between MMR and autism / inflammatory bowel disease?

- No clear link has been demonstrated between either autism or inflammatory bowel disease and MMR

---

### What are the contraindications to the MMR vaccine?

- Immunocompromised
- Malignancy
- Another live vaccine in the previous three weeks
- Acute febrile illness
- Gelatin or neomycin allergy

**1 //**   What side effects are associated with the MMR vaccine?

**2 //**   What is herd immunity, and how is this achieved?

**3 //**   How does measles typically present?

**4 //**   What are the complications of mumps?

**5 //**   How does rubella typically present?

# Station 7
# GENETIC COUNSELLING: CYSTIC FIBROSIS

*Candidate Briefing: Mr and Mrs Taylor are pregnant with their first child. They are concerned about cystic fibrosis, since Mrs Taylor's sister recently gave birth to a child with this condition. Please inform the couple about cystic fibrosis and advise them about their available options.*

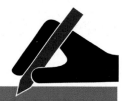

*Patient Briefing: You are Mrs Taylor, and are 5 weeks pregnant with your first child. Your sister recently gave birth to a child with cystic fibrosis, and they ended up going to intensive care with a severe chest infection. You know that it's a disease that runs in families. You are worried that your child will have it, and do not want to keep a child with what you perceive to be a major disability. You want to find out as early as possible whether this child has cystic fibrosis, as you would want a termination if the test for cystic fibrosis was positive.*

## Mark Scheme for Examiner

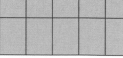

### Introduction

| | | | | |
|---|---|---|---|---|
| Cleans hands, introduces self, confirms patient identity | | | | |
| Establish current patient knowledge and concerns | | | | |

### Explaining Cystic Fibrosis

| | | | | |
|---|---|---|---|---|
| Defines CF, explains most commonly effected organs, and long term complications | | | | |
| Explains the concept of carrier for autosomal recessive disorder; ¼ risk of inheritance if both parents carrier | | | | |

Paediatrics

## Explain Testing

| | | | | | |
|---|---|---|---|---|---|
| Describes carrier testing | | | | | |
| Describes antenatal testing (chorionic villous sampling), and amniocentesis) with risks of miscarriage | | | | | |
| Describes neonatal testing | | | | | |

## Management of Cystic Fibrosis

| | | | | | |
|---|---|---|---|---|---|
| Possibility of termination | | | | | |
| Explains that although no known cure, multidisciplinary lifelong management | | | | | |

## Finishing the Consultation

| | | | | | |
|---|---|---|---|---|---|
| Elicit patient concerns or questions | | | | | |
| Summarise history back to parent | | | | | |
| Arrange a follow up appointment, offer your contact details | | | | | |
| Thank parent and close consultation | | | | | |

## General Points

| | | | | | |
|---|---|---|---|---|---|
| Check patient understands regularly, and offer information leaflets | | | | | |
| Maintain good eye contact | | | | | |
| Avoid medical jargon | | | | | |
| Polite to patient | | | | | |

**What is the inheritance pattern of cystic fibrosis?**

- Autosomal recessive

**What is the most common mutation that causes cystic fibrosis in Caucasion populations?**

- CFTR Delta 508 mutation

**Mrs Smith is a carrier for cystic fibrosis. Her partner does not have the disease, and is not a carrier. What are the chances of their child being a carrier, and what are the chances of their child having the disease?**

- The child has a 50% chance of being a carrier, but is extremely unlikely to have the disease (since their is no paternal copy of the gene to inherit)

**1 //** What are the respiratory complications of cystic fibrosis?

**2 //** What are the gastrointestinal complications of cystic fibrosis?

**3 //** What infection are people with CF particularly susceptible to?

**4 //** What is the typical life expectancy of someone with cystic fibrosis?

**5 //** How might cystic fibrosis present in a new born baby?

# Station 8
# GENETIC COUNSELLING: DOWN SYNDROME

*Candidate Briefing:* **Mr and Mrs Bradley are pregnant with their fourth child. They are concerned about the possibility of Down syndrome due to Mrs Bradley's age (35 years-old). Please advice the couple as to what Down syndrome is and what screening options are available.**

*Patient Briefing:* **You are Mr Bradley, and your wife is pregnant with your fourth child. She is 35 years old and you are concerned because of her age that you might have a child with Down syndrome. You know that this disease is associated with heart problems: a family friend had a child with Down syndrome, and they required major heart surgery to repair a hole in the heart. You are not sure whether this is a typical case of Down syndrome, and would like more information about the disease. You would want to keep the baby regardless of any diagnosis, but it is important for you to be able to plan parenthood in advance, and as early as possible, especially if this disease could be really severe.**

## Mark Scheme for Examiner

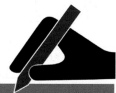

### Introduction

| | | | | |
|---|---|---|---|---|
| Cleans hands, introduces self, confirms patient identity | | | | |
| Establish current patient knowledge and concerns | | | | |

### Explaining Down Syndrome

| | | | | |
|---|---|---|---|---|
| Defines Down Syndrome, explains most commonly effected organs, and long term complications (heart, bowel, development) | | | | |

## Explain Testing

| | | | | | |
|---|---|---|---|---|---|
| Describes age related risk, and blood testing | | | | | |
| Describes definitive antenatal testing (chorionic villous sampling, and amniocentesis) with risks of miscarriage | | | | | |

## Management of Down Syndrome

| | | | | | |
|---|---|---|---|---|---|
| Possibility of termination | | | | | |
| Explains that although no known cure, multidisciplinary lifelong management of any problems | | | | | |

## Finishing the Consultation

| | | | | | |
|---|---|---|---|---|---|
| Elicit patient concerns or questions | | | | | |
| Summarise back to the patient | | | | | |
| Arrange a follow up appointment (as necessary) or offer your contact details | | | | | |
| Thank patient and close consultation | | | | | |

## General Points

| | | | | | |
|---|---|---|---|---|---|
| Check patient understands regularly, and offer information leaflets | | | | | |
| Maintain good eye contact | | | | | |
| Avoid medical jargon | | | | | |
| Polite to patient | | | | | |

## What is the genetic abnormality in Down syndrome?

- An additional copy of chromosome 21

## How might this be inherited?

- Trisomy 21 due to meiotic nondisjunction event in either male or female gamete
- Robertsonian translocation (the long arm of chromosome 21 is attached to another chromosome, often chromosome 14)
- Mosaic down syndrome: the meitoic nondisjunction event occurs after fertilization at some point during early cell division. Therefore these children have two cell lines: one with normal number of chromosomes (those cells unaffected), and one with an extra chromosome 21 (those cells affected)

## What are the most common cardiac complications of down syndrome?

- AVSD
- VSD

Paediatrics

**1 //** What are the typical facial features of the disease?

**2 //** What is the typical life expectancy of someone with Down syndrome?

**3 //** What blood tests can be done to screen for Down syndrome during pregnancy?

**4 //** What are the gastrointestinal complications of Down syndrome?

**5 //** Which malignancies are typically more likely in patients with Down syndrome?

# Station 9
# ASTHMA: PEAK FLOW

*Candidate Briefing: Mrs Patel has come to your clinic with her 7 year-old son, Sandeep. He has recently been diagnosed with asthma, and has been advised to keep a peak flow diary. Please teach him how to perform a peak flow.*

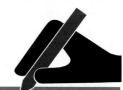

*Patient Briefing: You are a 7 year boy, who has never used a peak flow before. Assume no knowledge of using the peak flow, and follow the instructions of the doctor.*

## Mark Scheme for Examiner

### Introduction

| | | | | |
|---|---|---|---|---|
| Cleans hands, introduces self, confirms patient identity | | | | |
| Check identity of others in the room and confirm that the patient is happy for them to be present | | | | |
| Establish current patient knowledge and concerns | | | | |

### Explaining Peak Flow

| | | | | |
|---|---|---|---|---|
| Describes the technique of how to use the peak flow meter | | | | |
| Mentions that it must be done three times | | | | |
| Watches the patient do it without instruction | | | | |
| Show them how to use a peak flow diary | | | | |

Paediatrics

## Finishing the Consultation

| | | | | | |
|---|---|---|---|---|---|
| Elicit patient concerns or questions | | | | | |
| Summarise back to the patient | | | | | |
| Arrange a follow up appointment (as necessary) or offer your contact details | | | | | |
| Thank patient and close consultation | | | | | |

## General Points

| | | | | | |
|---|---|---|---|---|---|
| Check patient understands regularly, and offer information leaflets | | | | | |
| Maintain good eye contact and engage with patient | | | | | |
| Avoid medical jargon | | | | | |
| Polite to patient | | | | | |

## Questions And Answers for Candidate

### What peak flow (as a percentage of 'best') would make you concerned about life threatening asthma?

- <33%

### How might peak flow help in the diagnosis of chronic asthma?

- Demonstration of diurnal variation in peak flow of asthma
- May give clue as to environmental triggers in asthma

Paediatrics

## What are the typical changes on lung spirometry with asthma?

- There is an obstructive defect
- The FEV1 is reduced
- The FEV1 / FVC is reduced

## Additional Questions to Consider

**1 //**  What age group can peak flow be used for?

**2 //**  To get an accurate peak flow recording, how many times should you repeat it each time you record a peak flow?

**3 //**  If asthma was poorly controlled in a 7 year old, already on high dose inhaled steroids, and salbutamol as required, what would you consider next for treatment options?

**4 //**  When might absence of wheeze in the chest be a very poor sign in an asthmatic?

**5 //**  What is the hygiene hypothesis, and how does this relate to the increasing incidence of asthma?

Paediatrics

# Station 10
# ASTHMA: INHALER TECHNIQUE

*Candidate Briefing: Mrs Andrews has come to your clinic with her son James, aged 8 years. He has recently been diagnosed with asthma, and has commenced using regular inhalers. Please teach them how to use an inhaler with a spacer.*

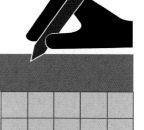

*Patient Briefing: You are an 8 year boy, who has never used an inhaler / spacer before. Assume no knowledge of using the inhaler/spacer, and follow the instructions of the doctor.*

## Mark Scheme for Examiner

### Introduction

| | | | | |
|---|---|---|---|---|
| Cleans hands, introduces self, confirms patient identity | | | | |
| Check identity of others in the room and confirm that the patient is happy for them to be present | | | | |
| Establish current patient knowledge and concerns | | | | |
| Explains the difference between blue and brown inhaler | | | | |

### Explaining Meter Dose Inhaler

| | | | | |
|---|---|---|---|---|
| Describes the technique of how to use the meter dose inhaler (with or without spacer depending on what is available in the exam) | | | | |
| Mentions that the inhaler has an expiry date, and lasts around 200 puffs; talk about how to wash and when to replace a spacer | | | | |
| Watches the patient do it without instruction | | | | |

Paediatrics

## Finishing the Consultation

| | | | | | |
|---|---|---|---|---|---|
| Elicit patient concerns or questions | | | | | |
| Summarise back to the patient | | | | | |
| Arrange a follow up appointment (as necessary) or offer your contact details | | | | | |
| Thank patient and close consultation | | | | | |

## General Points

| | | | | | |
|---|---|---|---|---|---|
| Check patient understands regularly, and offer information leaflets | | | | | |
| Maintain good eye contact | | | | | |
| Avoid medical jargon | | | | | |
| Polite to patient | | | | | |

## Questions And Answers for Candidate

### What are the common side effects of inhaled steroids?

- Hoarseness to the voice
- Oral candida infection

Paediatrics

> **In terms of the frequency of use of salbutamol, when should a parent be advised to seek medical review for their child?**

- If using it more than 3 times a week, or if needing more than 6 puffs in one go

## Additional Questions to Consider

**1 //** How long can a spacer be used for?

**2 //** How do you wash a spacer, and how often is this needed?

**3 //** What are the advantages of using a spacer?

**4 //** If inhaled low dose steroids and salbutamol as required are not sufficient to control the asthma in an eight year old, what might you consider next?

**5 //** What environmental factors might contribute to poor asthma control?